THE ART OF
EROTIC
MASSAGE

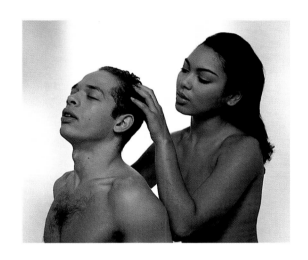

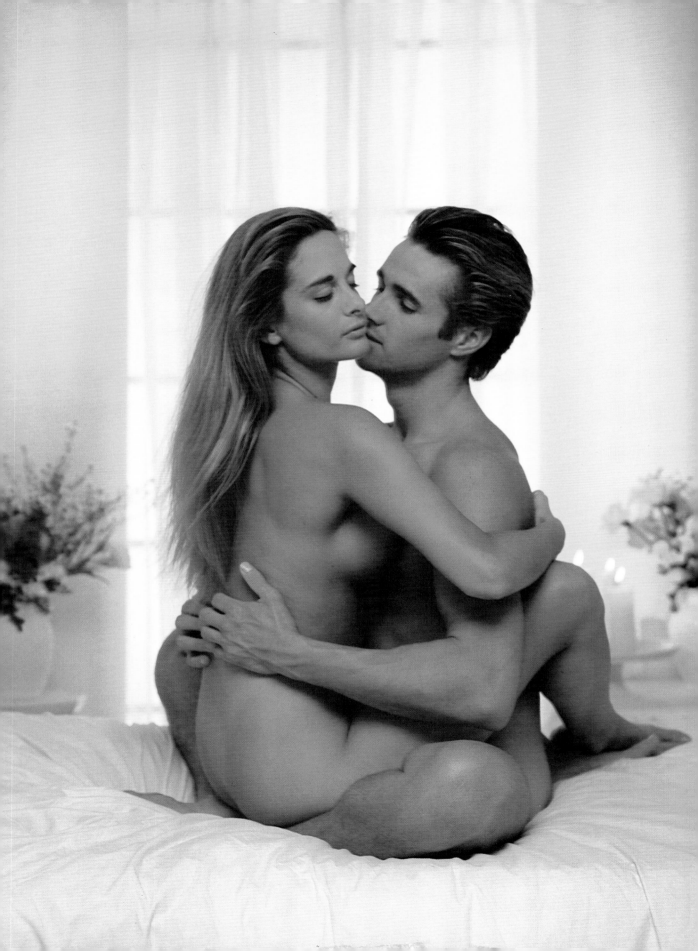

The Art of
Erotic
MASSAGE

NITYA LACROIX

PHOTOGRAPHED BY ALAN RANDALL

To Mary Ling for her friendship and inspiration

PRODUCED BY CARLTON BOOKS

This edition published in 1994 by
Virgin Books
an imprint of Virgin Publishing Ltd
332 Ladbroke Grove
London W10 5AH

Text and Design Copyright © 1994 Carlton Books Limited

A CIP catalogue record for this book is available from the British Library

ISBN 0 86369-845-X

Aromatherapy recipes provided by Sakina Bowhay

Project Art Director: Bobbie Colgate-Stone
Design: Alison Kyles
Project Executive Editors: Lorraine Dickey and Tessa Rose
Production: Garry Lewis

Printed and bound in Italy

Contents

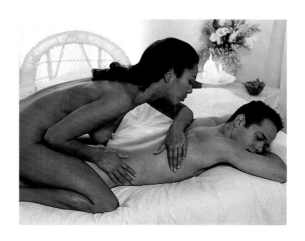

The language of touch

The human body has a tremendous capacity to experience pleasure through its five senses: sight, sound, smell, taste and, above all, touch. Heightening these senses to the point of exquisite joy is a playful art which brings a new and deeper level of intimacy between two people in a loving relationship. Massage is a means through which two people in an intimate relationship can help each other relax and explore the realms of sensuality and eroticism.

TOUCH, IT IS SAID, is food for our souls, and the tactile experience is essential for the development of wholesome, happy people. Many eminent psychologists believe that touch deprivation in childhood is one of the root causes of neurosis and unsociable behaviour. In fact, a huge part of our brain is given over to the sensory and tactile department. Touch is the primary sense we develop, the first one that an embryo experiences within the womb as it strokes its thumb or finger across its skin. For a newborn baby, touch is the first point of contact with a strange new world as it is cradled against the warmth and comfort of its mother's skin. It is through being touched with love that we establish our self-esteem and appreciation for our own bodies. These attitudes, developed early in our lives, play a large part in creating a happy and fulfilling sexual relationship.

Loving touch within massage will enrich the sensual and emotional aspect of your relationship.

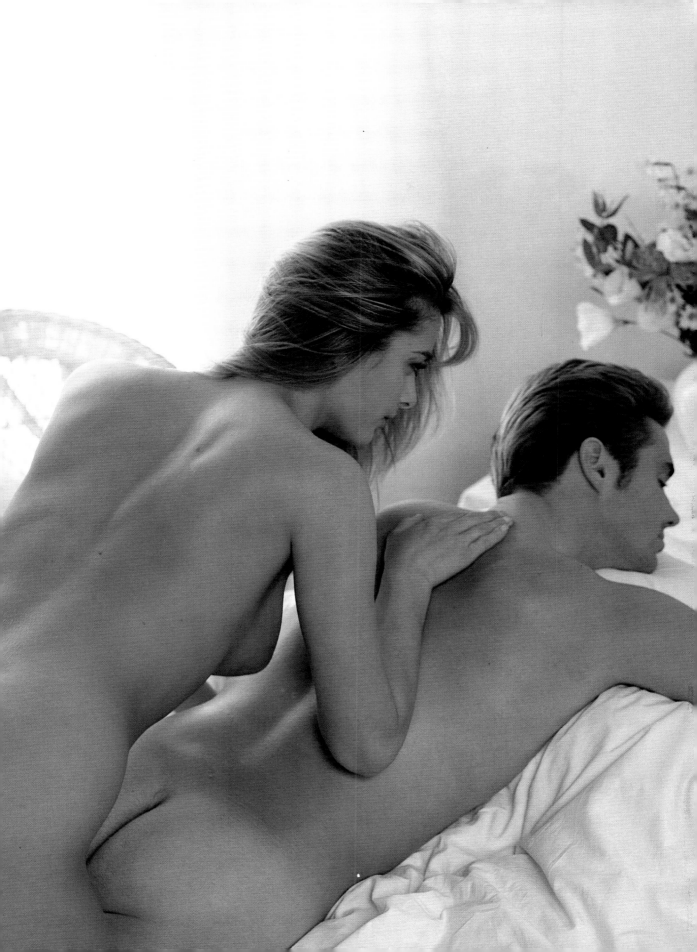

The longing to be touched remains with us as adults, all the more so if we lacked tactile contact in childhood. Promiscuity is often a search for simple loving touch and a need to be nurtured, though in seeking satisfaction from meaningless sexual relationships a person may become unhappy and frustrated. Sadly, the mysteries of pleasuring one another through loving touch and massage have been greatly neglected, and the body's more subtle senses are relatively ignored. Aggressive visual and aural sensations dominate in many cultures, so that the more delicate levels of sensual awareness and receptivity have become dulled. Touch, the body and pleasure have been too often subjected to moral condemnation or relegated to the sex industry to be exploited for image and profit. Even within a sexual relationship, the exploration of the senses and the language of touch, which can set alight the whole body, may be lost when sex becomes a purely genital experience with orgasm and ejaculation the only goal in mind.

Women are generally more 'in touch' with their overall sensuality than men and love to be shown through touch that they are appreciated in ways other than just for their sexuality. Men tend to be more sexually focused in a physical relationship, but once they discover the delights of full body sensuality, they are readily converted. By learning the art and skills of massage, both partners have the opportunity to give and receive whole body pleasure.

All of our senses, particularly our skin responses, are the bridge between the outer realities of life and our internal experiences of them. Touch, skin and feelings are inextricable from one another. To be touched with love and to have our skin caressed with tenderness nurtures the deeper levels of our being. Without words, the calm, still presence of the hands upon the body will reassure and relax the mind and the emotions. The skin, the largest organ of the body, is alive with millions of sensory cells and receptors, relaying messages to the brain through a complex network of nerves. Let the message of love, appreciation and joy come from your fingertips onto the skin of your loved one to bring alive sensuality and sheer pleasure simply for its own sake.

THE STROKES OF MASSAGE

The following strokes form the basic techniques of a soft-tissue massage to help you and your lover enrich your relationship through the communication of touch. If the mood of the massage is extremely sensuous you may want to keep your strokes soft and flowing, using the flat of your hands to caress, slither and slide all over the body. However, even during a very tender and loving massage, your partner may appreciate the addition of more invigorating techniques such as kneading. It is important that you blend the relaxing and revitalizing strokes together in a harmonious way. Play between the two types of movements, allowing one motion to merge into another as if you were creating a harmonious symphony of music on your partner's body. Let your strokes be fluid and never jerky, and always take them around or out of the body rather than stopping them abruptly in mid-flow.

Here are some of the various styles of strokes that will make your massage satisfying, soothing and beneficial.

SENSUAL, RELAXING STROKES

Always begin massaging an area of the body with the softer, more sensual strokes to relax your partner psychologically as well as physically, and to warm up and stretch the body's soft tissue.

Here are a selection of strokes which will begin to soothe your partner.

1. Fan strokes

Fan strokes can be applied all over the body and vary in size depending on the particular effect you are wishing to achieve. Smaller fan strokes applied with a degree of pressure and moving up the body stretch tissue and release tension from the muscles in addition to boosting the blood circulation towards the heart. Larger, softer fan strokes have a more relaxing and euphoric effect. These flowing fan strokes should slide over the skin at a steady pressure from the full surface of the hands. When you are enlarging them to encompass the contours of an area of the body, your hands should be sufficiently soft to melt and mould into the shape of the body.

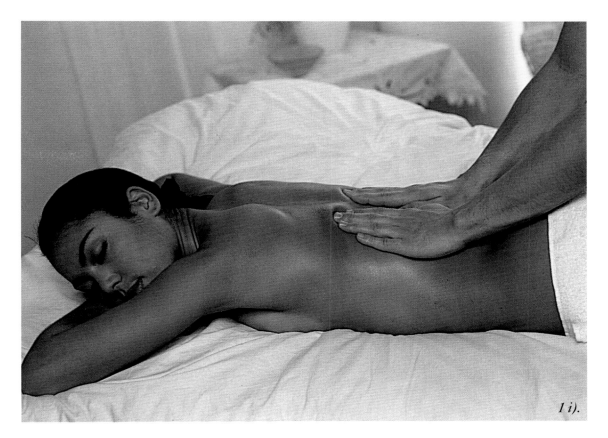

1 i).

1 i). Place both hands close together alongside the spine so they rest flat on the body with the fingers pointing towards the head. Begin to stroke firmly and steadily upwards for about 15cm/6 inches, distributing the pressure evenly through the hands.

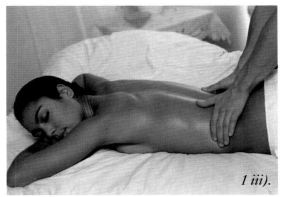

1 iii).

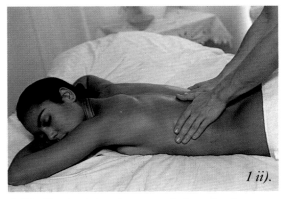

1 ii).

1 ii). Fan both hands outwards in a circular arc so that your fingers embrace the sides of the body as they glide back down.

1 iii). Swivel your wrists so that both hands sweep together at a lighter pressure back in towards the

initial source of the stroke. Glide them a short distance up the body and, without halting the motion, begin the next fan stroke. When your fan strokes reach the top of the shoulders or limbs sweep your hands in a rounded movement over each side of the body area to encompass its shape, and glide back down the sides to where the strokes began. A fan stroke sequence can be repeated three times on any area of the body for a fully relaxing effect to prepare for more invigorating strokes.

2. Circle strokes

Circle strokes are soothing and excellent for stretching the body's soft tissue. Use them on the back, front and sides of the body. In this movement, only the left hand makes a complete circle, while the right hand makes a half-circle. Use the circles to stroke over the skin in a constant flowing movement.

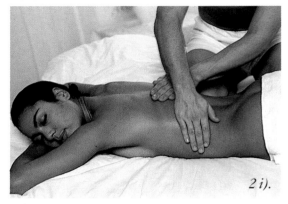

2 i).

2 i). Rest both hands parallel and flat on the body, fingers pointing away from you. Begin to slide both hands into a circular motion.

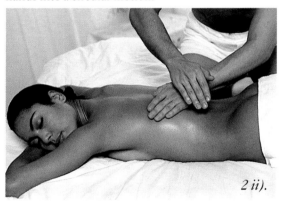

2 ii).

2 ii). As the left hand makes the first arc of the circle, your right hand lifts off the body to allow it to circle over the skin. The right hand crosses over the top of the left hand and drops lightly back down onto the body. As the left hand completes the full circular motion the right hand performs a semi-circular motion, retracing the movement of the left hand before lifting up off the body again.

3. Stretches

As your hands skate over the body, they can spread apart to cover areas such as the back and the legs at the same time and then slide together, so the effect is of many hands stroking and loving the body. This freewheeling effect on the skin is guaranteed to bring your partner out of his head and into his body as he surrenders himself to the sensation of an all-encompassing touch. Stretch strokes are wonderful movements that bring a feeling of length, expansion, body integration and release of tension. Vary the pressure in your hands so that it is firmer as they move apart and softer as they glide back towards each other. The sensation you want to create is that of stretching the tissue outwards rather than pushing it back in towards the centre of the body.

3 i). Mould your hands into the body shape as they move out from the centre of the back, one hand stroking towards the shoulder while the other moves towards the leg diagonally opposite. Use the flat of your hands, your forearms or as much of your

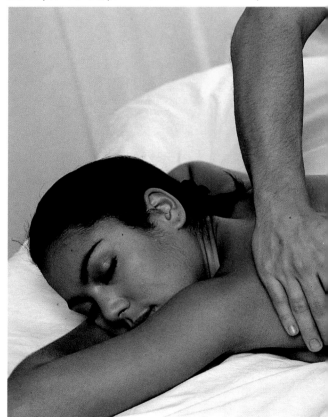

own body as is comfortably possible, to make skin to skin contact.

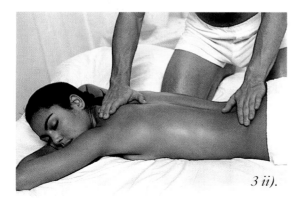

3 ii).

3 ii). Back stretches bring a sense of relief to a tense area. Place both hands flat, with fingers pointing away from you, on the centre of the spine. Pressure on the spine must always be light. Draw both hands over the spine in opposite directions, one stroking up towards the neck and over the head while the other moves down towards the base. Rest both hands quietly over these areas to make a calming

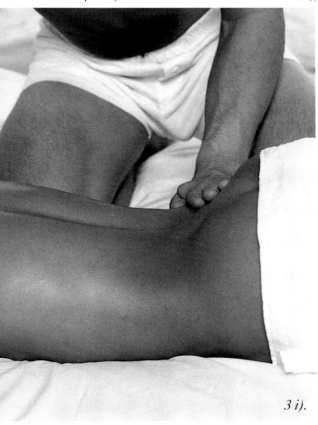

3 i).

contact before bringing your hands back to the centre of the spine. Now stroke your hands firmly out in diagonally opposite directions so that one moves towards the shoulder and the other towards the opposite hip. Lightly slide back to the centre of the spine and stroke both hands out to embrace the other hip and shoulder.

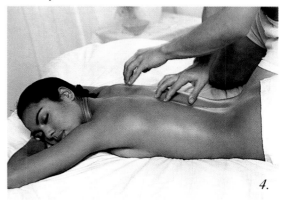

4.

4. Raking touches
Raking is excellent to use after a sequence of massage strokes to stimulate nerve endings close to the surface of the skin and to bring a sense of directing tension release out of the body. Let your hands become slightly claw-shaped and use your fingertips to rake over the skin in short, overlapping movements, one hand following the other in a consistent downward motion. Rake from the top to the end of the limb or body area.

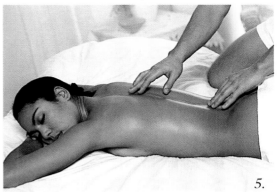

5.

5. Feathering
Soften your hands and use the fingertips to stroke with the lightest of touches down the body in the same fashion as the raking movements. Feathering is particularly sensual and sends thrilling shivers through the body.

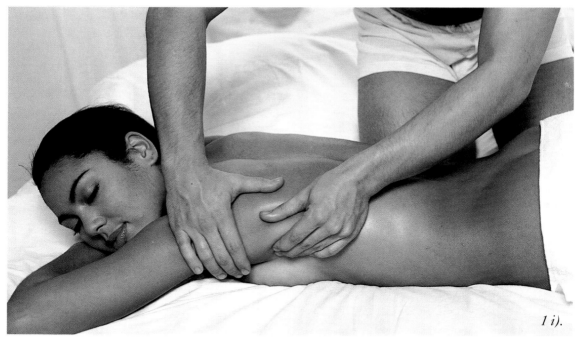

1 i).

REVITALIZING STROKES
1 i). Kneading

Kneading should be applied after muscles have been soothed and warmed by sensual strokes. Follow up kneading with soft strokes. Kneading works best when applied in a constant rhythmic motion, with relaxed wrists and firm, rounded movements. Its action should resemble the hand movements of a baker kneading dough and its benefits include invigoration, relaxation, and the breaking down and removal of fatty deposits and toxins from the tissues. Kneading creates a satisfying feeling that the muscles are being firmly held and moved and it certainly has its place in a sensual massage, particularly when applied over fleshy areas such as the thighs and buttocks.

1 ii). Use your right hand to lift, squeeze and roll the flesh towards your left hand. Your left hand then takes the flesh and repeats the action by rolling it back to the right hand.

2. Pressure strokes

Pressure strokes push steadily down on the flesh by the focusing of weight into distinct areas of your hands, such as fingertips, thumbpads and heels, to remove a deeper level of tension from tight muscles. Apply them only when the body tissues have been thoroughly warmed and soothed by other movements.

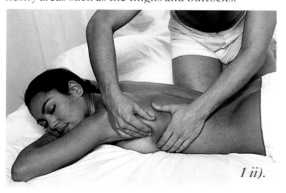

1 ii).

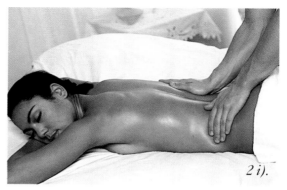

2 i).

2 i). Alternating fan strokes

These strokes use the whole surface of the hands but pressure is applied specifically on the movement of the heels and sides of the thumbs while the fingers simultaneously stroke around and back down the sides of the body part. The hands, one following the other, fan out in alternating motions up over the area before gliding more softly back down and in towards the next stroke. Apply them to the legs, arms and lower back after softer strokes and kneading.

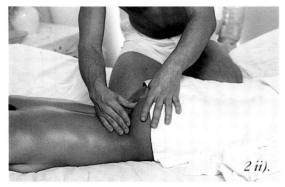

2 ii).

2 ii). Thumb-pressure strokes

Rotate the thumb joints and apply pressure into the thumbpads so that one follows another in small, alternating circles over an area of muscle. Both hands should rest on the body to support the movement of the stroke. Once you have reached the top of the area you are immediately massaging, glide both hands back down to repeat the sequence or move into the next stroke.

3. Vibratory strokes

By moving both hands in rapid succession on the fleshy surface of the skin you can stimulate your partner, boost the blood circulation, tone up the muscles and leave the body glowing. Keep your shoulders and wrists relaxed as you apply these strokes and quickly flick your hands off the skin to

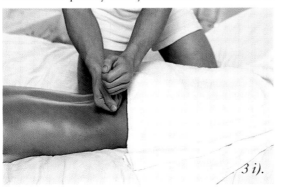

3 i).

achieve a percussion effect. These strokes bring an enlivening finish to your massage as you complete a sequence on a specific area. Follow them up with raking or feathering touches.

3 i). Pummelling

Make loose fists and briskly pummel the flesh with the sides of both hands following each other in quick succession. Use pummelling on the thighs, buttocks and shoulders.

3 ii). Hacking

Keep both hands open, with fingers relaxed and close together. Using the sides of the hands, strike the skin in fast vibratory motions, one hand following the other.

WHEN TO SEEK ADVICE ABOUT MASSAGE

Massage has many therapeutic values, whether its aim is for pure pleasure, relaxation or invigoration. There are some occasions and conditions, however, when it is not a suitable treatment. If your partner is being treated for a medical condition, always seek medical advice. Cardio-vascular diseases, including thrombosis, phlebitis, oedema and heart disease, are contra-indicated to massage. Never massage directly over skin infections, septic areas such as boils, inflammation, undiagnosed lumps, recent scar tissue or varicose veins. Avoid giving massage when a person has a fever, high temperature or a heavy cold as the body is already working hard to eliminate toxins or foreign bodies. Consult a doctor in cases of cancer, Aids, epilepsy, psychiatric illnesses, frailty or pregnancy.

Remember, if you are in doubt as to the suitability of massage, always seek proper medical advice.

If you plan to use aromatherapy oils, it is very important to bear in mind that essential oils are extremely potent and should be diluted strictly according to the instructions given by a qualified aromatherapist. Never ingest aromatherapy oils internally. If you are in any doubt as to the correct usage of the oils or their suitability always seek the advice of a qualified practitioner, particularly when you are working with conditions such as pregnancy, frailty, Aids, cancer, epilepsy, heart or cardiovascular problems, allergies and skin ailments.

Relaxation
& invigoration

Stress can be one of the main culprits for sapping your vitality and health and robbing you of your sexual energy. Even the happiest relationships are vulnerable to its insidious effects. Stress build-up causes tension in both the body and mind which, unresolved, can disturb an easy, open communication and a satisfying sex life between a loving couple.

ONE OF THE BEST ways of discharging stress and staying happy and healthy is by enjoying good sex – a fact that has been endorsed not only over recent years by eminent Western sex therapists but, according to ancient manuscripts, was strongly advocated thousands of years ago by Chinese scholars and physicians.

However, a good sex life does not happen automatically. Once the first flush of passion subsides, sustaining a fulfilling sexual relationship requires the on-going attention of the two people involved, to both their own needs and each other's. Sex at its best is not only a whole body experience, but a whole person experience. Body and mind are both involved and so too are the emotional vulnerabilities of both people. Stress will have an effect on all these areas, causing conscious and unconscious tensions which will inhibit physical and emotional relaxation between the couple.

A certain amount of stress is a natural part of life and is essential to keep you alert, motivated and able to respond to stimuli. Certain emotions such as anger, fear, excitement and anxiety activate your 'fight or flight' responses, sending signals to the brain so that hormones such as adrenalin and cortisol

Creating time within your relationship to help each other to relax will directly benefit your loving and intimate communication.

14

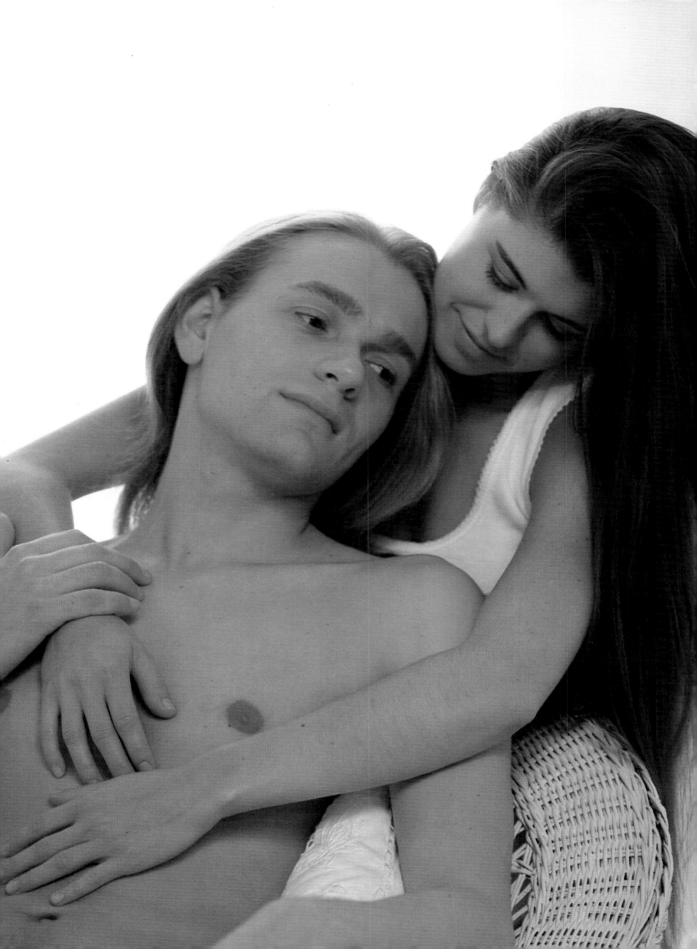

are released into the blood, increasing your heart rate, metabolism and blood pressure and generally empowering you to respond physically to a stressful situation. Unfortunately, the fast pace of modern life does not always allow you the opportunity to discharge your stress; instead, you hold it pent up within your body. Prolonged stress depletes you of your vitality, lowers your immune system's resistance to infection, and can cause a number of stress-related conditions such as depression, lethargy, hypertension, ulcers and muscular aches and pains. It also plays havoc with your love-life. If at the end of the day you feel tense, tired or anxious you might perceive your loved one's sexual desire for you as just one more unwanted demand on your time and attention. Stress and its related effects are some of the most common causes of impotence in men and lack of sexual response in women.

THE IMPORTANCE OF MASSAGE

Massage is now recognized as one of the most beneficial therapies for stress. It is a powerful skill to learn if you are part of a loving couple, not only because its tactile and sensuous uses can enhance the eroticism of your love-making, but also because it helps to alleviate the basic physical and emotional tensions that can build up, inhibiting a relaxed communication between you and your partner.

You do not need to be a qualified massage therapist to give a wonderfully relaxing or invigorating massage to your partner. If you trust your hands, and you touch your lover with care and empathy, the very quality of that loving contact will help to release tensions, soothe the mind, and bring you closer together.

Massage is fun to give and delightful to receive, and it can be a relaxing event for both people at the same time. Once you feel confident about giving massage, you will probably find that your hands are almost itching to get into those tight nooks and crannies of your partner's body. However, it is important that you only give massage when you want to or you will find that your resentment will sneak its way through your hands into your strokes.

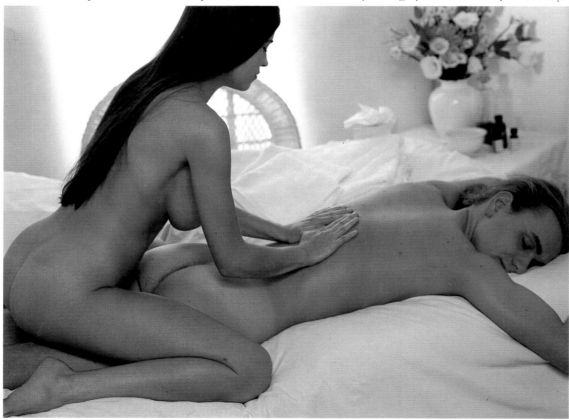

HOW IT WORKS

Massage works in many different ways. Touch is a non-verbal language all of its own which does not contain the pressure of more direct mental communication. It allows time to unwind, to get back in contact with your body and to let go of stressful thoughts and physical aches and pains. It creates a welcome space between the pressures of daily life and the need to just relax and enjoy the pleasure of physical and mental intimacy.

A comforting touch and light stroking of the skin has a direct effect on the nervous system which can produce a soporific feeling of emotional well-being. Other massage techniques have direct physiological and psychological effects. Massage strokes warm and relax tight, tense muscles by stretching soft tissue, boosting the circulation system, helping the exchange of tissue fluids and removing the body's waste products caught in muscle fibres. Performed softly, the strokes relax and replenish vital energy: applied deeper or more vigorously, they can invigorate and stimulate the whole physical system, clear the mind, and help you acknowledge and let go of negative emotions. Being touched is a nurturing experience which helps to relieve the sense of isolation that stress creates. In this way, massage works on the whole person.

HOW TO PREPARE FOR MASSAGE

While you are giving your partner a massage he or she will be sitting or lying still, so you need to ensure that the room is warm and draught-free. Even the most basic massage programmes work better if you are not interrupted and you have some privacy so that you can dedicate yourselves totally to each other.

Always make sure that both you and your partner are positioned comfortably during a massage. The last thing you should do is give a lovely relaxing massage but end up suffering from stiff shoulders or

Tender touch combined with skilful massage strokes can enliven the spirit while at the same time bringing ease to the body and mind.

an aching back. Tips to remember about your own posture while giving massage are to make sure you are always breathing fully, and that your spine, shoulders, arms, wrists and hands are relaxed at all times. Adding pressure to a massage stroke is done by applying your body weight, not by muscle power. Always remember that the more comfortable you are in giving a massage the more relaxed your partner will become.

APPLYING OIL

In order to lubricate the skin and give your strokes a sensuous feel, you should use a little oil or lotion. You can buy specially prepared massage oils from health shops and chemists, or you can use baby oil or a good-quality light vegetable oil such as grapeseed or safflower. You can add a few drops of a richer oil such as almond, avocado or wheatgerm for a more luxuriant effect. Place a few drops of oil into the palms of your hands and warm it by rubbing your hands together before spreading it over the skin. Apply just enough oil to the skin to allow a smooth glide of your hands – too much oil will make the skin slippery and prevent your hands from working deeper into the muscles, while too little can cause your strokes to burn the skin.

If you or your partner do not like the feeling of oil on the skin you can use talcum powder, but this will prevent you performing some of the more flowing strokes.

THE MASSAGE PROGRAMMES

This chapter presents three simple massage programmes for relaxation and invigoration which are focused on the main tension areas in the body. Use them on each other at the end of a tiring or stressful day, whenever you need a boost of energy, or when you feel that tactile contact will be the best and most loving form of communication between you.

Take turns in giving each other massage, focusing on the areas which most require attention. For instance, one of you can receive a relaxing shoulder and neck massage before the other then enjoys a pampering hand massage. Alternatively, simply devote time to your partner knowing that the favour will be returned when you are in need.

UP TO YOUR NECK IN IT

More than in any other part of the body, you are most likely to feel tension in the shoulders and neck – ask anyone where they experience stiffness or pain and they nearly always point to this area. Sometimes the pain results from habitual tension caused by holding and moving the body in a certain way, or it may arise from sitting for prolonged periods hunched over a desk. More often than not it is a temporary discomfort resulting from added emotional stress. Tightening the shoulders seems to be a natural physical mechanism of protection when the going gets rough and a way of warding off difficult situations and uncomfortable feelings. Tensing the neck and contracting the muscles around the shoulders is a bit like trying to force a wedge between the irresistible force of feelings and the immovable object of mind. We do it whenever we are upset or under stress in order to prevent ourselves from expressing emotions that we might judge inappropriate in the circumstances. Note what happens when you are stuck in a traffic jam – your shoulders go up, your jaw tightens and your hands grip the wheel. When any unpleasant aspects of your life become overwhelming, the world seems to sit on your shoulders. Tensing and contracting the muscles is usually an unconscious response, and if you do not catch it in time and learn to release it this response builds up to the point where it can cause chronic pain and discomfort.

Unfortunately, just as the tension blocks your expression of negative feelings in a difficult situation, so it may inhibit your relaxation and spontaneity when you most want to express your warmth and affection to the person you love. In fact, you bring the tension home with you, locked up in your shoulders and neck. You may then perpetuate your discomfort by being unable to respond to the very person you love and who could do the most to return you to a feeling of relaxation.

So, learn to use this easy 15-minute shoulder and neck massage programme, combined with some body awareness techniques, as part of the many routine ways in which you express your caring for each other. It will bring swift relief to a tense body and restore ease to the mind. Both of you will benefit!

MASSAGE FOR THE RELIEF OF SHOULDER AND NECK TENSION

Relief of the superficial causes of shoulder and neck pain can be achieved quite quickly in this short massage. The strokes can be adapted to work well on tense shoulder muscles while your partner is still wearing clothes, so privacy is not an essential requirement. However, the massage is more effective when applied to bare skin because then you can add some lubrication to your hands and apply the more flowing strokes which will warm, soften and ease the muscles.

This massage will be more comfortable for your partner if you ask her to straddle a chair so that she faces its back. She can lean forward into the support of a pillow for comfort. Never try to force or hurry someone into relaxation, as this will feel like added pressure. It takes time to let tensions dissolve, so start with some verbal suggestions for relaxation that will help your partner bring some self-awareness back to her body and encourage her to feel more at ease in her posture. Stress commonly causes people to focus on their mental energies so that the connection with their physical feelings is neglected. This leads to a sense of being 'uprooted' and without solid foundation. An awareness of the body and breathing at all times helps to stabilize both mind and emotions, particularly in times of crisis and anxiety. Gently suggest to your partner that she take some moments to allow her feet to relax on the ground. This is useful in helping her 'come down to earth', particularly if she is feeling stressed or mentally over-active.

Next, suggest to your partner that she moves around on the chair until she feels her pelvis is properly supporting the upper half of her body, taking the strain off her lower back. Ask her to take three deep breaths into her belly to help her relax her whole body. Give her an image to use which suggests the tension held around her spine, shoulders and neck is melting each time she exhales. If her shoulder joints feel particularly stiff, ask her to draw them up as she breathes in and drop them down with the out-breath three times. She should then wriggle her arms, wrists, hands and fingers around freely as if to shake out the remaining tensions.

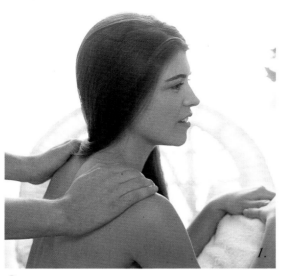

GIVING THE MASSAGE

1. Stand behind your partner and rest your hands softly over each shoulder. This is a hold which will give her time to relax into the warmth and contact of your touch. After a stressful day, the caring, gentle presence of your hands on her shoulders will reassure her and help bring her attention to this area of her body, so that she can start to unwind.

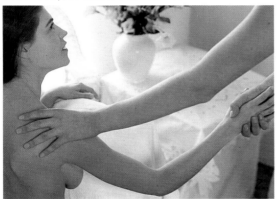

2. Begin with passive movements which will help to relax the shoulder joints and arms. Stand just in front and facing your partner's right shoulder. Place your left hand lightly over it and clasp her hand in your right hand. Encourage your partner to let the whole weight of her arm drop and to allow you to make all the movements. Keeping her elbow flexed, extend her arm away from her body and rock it gently and rhythmically back and forth and up and down. The more confidence you display in your hands with the movement, the more she will be able

to relax the weight of her arm and consequently the tightness in her shoulder. Now repeat these passive movements on the left side of her body.

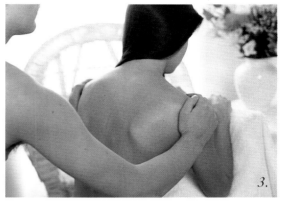

3. Stand behind your partner and rub a little oil or lotion into your hands, then begin to spread it with soft, flowing movements around the mid-to-upper back, shoulders and upper arms. These stroking motions will begin to warm and relax the area, easing away stiffness from tense tissue. Let your hands fan out, encircle and define the rounded shape of the shoulders, shoulder blades and sides of the body.

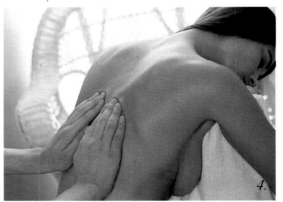

4. Ask your partner to lean forward into the pillow. Place both of your hands, fingers pointing towards her head, on each side of her spine about mid-back. Steadily glide your hands up alongside her spine to give the long muscles on each side a good stretch. In a continuous movement, draw your hands outwards over her shoulders to the top of her arms, and then pull them firmly back down along the sides of the ribcage. Glide your hands lightly back to where you began your stroke and repeat this movement about five times without breaking the sequence.

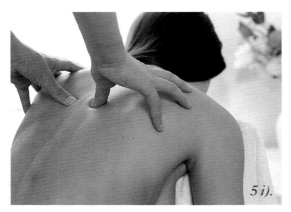

5 i).

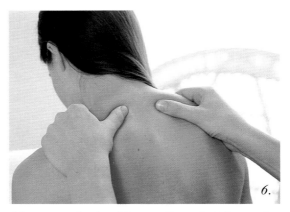

6.

5 i). A loose, flexible spine keeps both body and mind feeling fit and healthy. Ease tense spots by working your way up each side of the spine with thumb pad pressure. Lean your body weight into your thumbs while resting your fingers on her back. The secret to success with this movement is to add and release the pressure slowly and to check with your partner to ensure the pressure feels comfortable. Move up her spine about an inch at a time, spending a few seconds on each point.

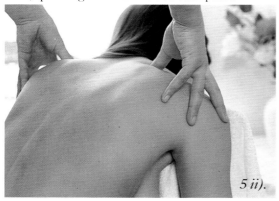

5 ii).

5 ii). Continue this thumb pressure along the muscle across the top of her shoulders. Now soothe the whole area again with a sequence of flowing strokes.

6. By now, the upper back should be warm and relaxed enough for some more invigorating work. Begin by kneading both shoulders. Anchor the fingers of both hands over the shoulders and using the heels and sides of your thumbs, roll and squeeze the fleshy area upwards. Keep your fingers resting over the shoulders and release the pressure in your hands to glide them lightly in a circle back into a position where they can repeat the stroke. Work in

this way on the shoulders until you feel the tension melting. Now squeeze and knead the flesh down the top of both arms, using one hand on each side. Follow up the kneading motions with a sequence of flowing strokes.

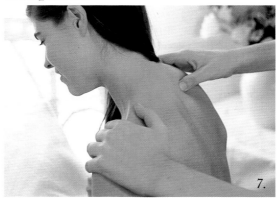

7.

7. While you are working on the shoulders, your hands might discover little areas of knotted tissue which are usually quite painful. These are normally caused by deposits of waste products trapped in tight muscle. Some grinding movements will help to disperse them back into the body's natural elimination system and consequently bring greater relief to the whole area. Place your hands in the same position as with the previous kneading stroke, but this time work in small circles with pressure from your thumb pads, working on one spot at a time all around the area between the shoulder blade and spine and at the base of the neck. Work both thumbs simultaneously, and then increase your pressure by working with one thumb on one side at a time. Help to boost the elimination of toxins and increase the blood circulation to the area by a series of firm, flowing strokes.

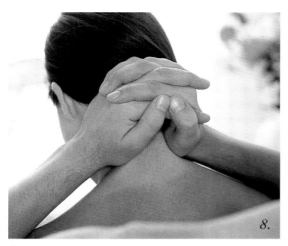

8.

8. By now your partner's shoulders will be relaxing, but attention must be given to her neck and head. Ask her to lean her head forward a little to stretch her neck. Lightly clasp your fingers together, and work from the base of the neck to the edge of the skull and back by sliding the heels of your hands in a continuous upward-moving rotation, giving a little squeeze to the neck muscle as your hands move inwards. Be careful here not to inadvertently pull your partner's hair.

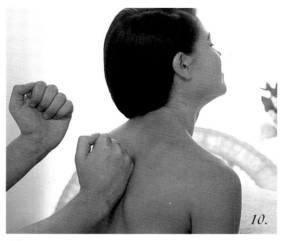

10.

10. Having relaxed her shoulders and neck, give your partner a vigorous boost with some percussion movements over her shoulders and alongside her spine. Relax your wrists and make loose fists. Pummel gently but briskly, one hand following the other, across the top of her shoulders and beside her shoulder blades, flicking the edge of your hands off the skin as soon as they make contact. Make sure that you do not strike the spine or other bony areas as this will cause discomfort.

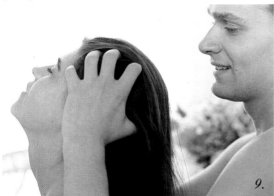

9.

9. Now use your fingertips to massage thoroughly in small circles all over your partner's scalp to release that uncomfortable sense of pressure in the head which results from stress. Your hands should be slightly claw-shaped to add reasonable pressure into your fingers. Work on one area at a time so that you can feel the scalp move.

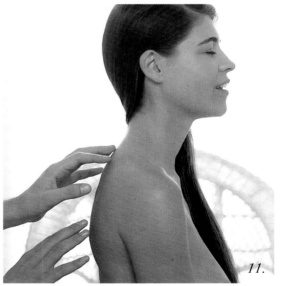

11.

11. Complete your shoulder and neck massage with delightful, soft, feather-like touches of your fingertips to bring a tingle to the skin and stimulate its senses. Run your fingertips in light, flowing strokes first down the neck and across the shoulders, then down the back.

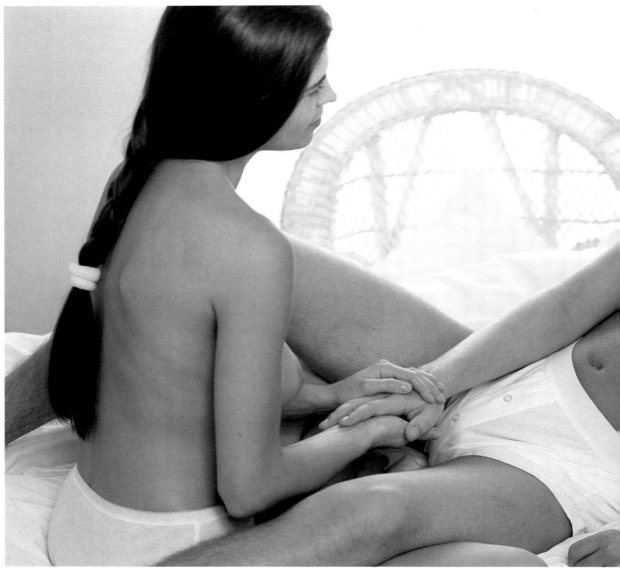

TAKING HOLD OF THE HANDS

The fact that we human beings can use our hands to grasp, clutch, stroke and mould has played a huge part in our successful evolution and survival. A number of psychologists have pointed out that there is a definite link between hand dexterity and greater intellect.

Our hands are highly sensitive and are intricate in their constitution. Each contains 27 small bones and thousands of nerve endings which relay messages to and from the brain. In fact, the part of the brain allotted to receiving and imparting messages from and to the thumbs and fingers is proportionately one of its largest areas. Movement happens in the fingers through the action of muscles in the forearm which are attached to the finger bones by long tendons running through the back of the hand – so when you want to massage the hand and help to reduce stiffness, remember to include the forearm in your strokes.

If your partner is involved in work that requires repetitive hand, wrist and arm movement, such as using a keyboard, a tool, a driving wheel or a musical instrument, a considerable amount of tension could be building up in the hand and arm. This can also create an underlying level of psychological stress.

comfort, solidarity, love and companionship. Hands symbolically express our capacity to give and receive. We reach out with our hands to explore the world around us, defining through the sense of touch our outer reality to our inner perceptions. Hands so often express our inner emotions: clenched and tense they portray anger; cold and trembling they expose fear, excitement or anticipation; warm and relaxed they are capable of expressing our innermost feelings of tenderness and love through the gentlest of caresses. When we see something that evokes our personal sense of beauty or kindness, we spontaneously reach out to touch it with our hands. So take your partner's hands into your own, and let this hand massage be a loving gesture that allows both a physical relaxation and an emotional intimacy.

The beauty of a hand massage is that it is so simple to do. It does not require special preparation and even a 10-minute massage on each hand and forearm can work wonders. As a special treat, use a specially formulated hand lotion which moisturizes and softens the skin at the same time as your massage helps to keep the hand supple. Both of you should be sitting comfortably, well propped up by cushions if necessary. Keep checking that your partner's arm is well supported and the elbow joint remains relaxed.

THE HAND MASSAGE

1. The first thing to do is to hold your partner's hand softly cupped between your own. The warmth and presence of your hands will offer a comforting message of relaxation, allowing the muscles and tendons the time to relax. You are giving the hand permission simply 'to be' rather than 'to do'. Holding the hand imparts that universal signal of caring and will allow an empathetic exchange of feeling between the two of you so that the relaxation will happen on both a physical and emotional level.

2. Begin your strokes by connecting the hand to the forearm with sweeping and gliding motions that move from the wrist to the elbow and back again. At the same time, you will warm and stretch the forearm muscles, boosting the blood circulation up the arm. Rub some lotion into your hands and clasp your partner's right hand with your own right hand.

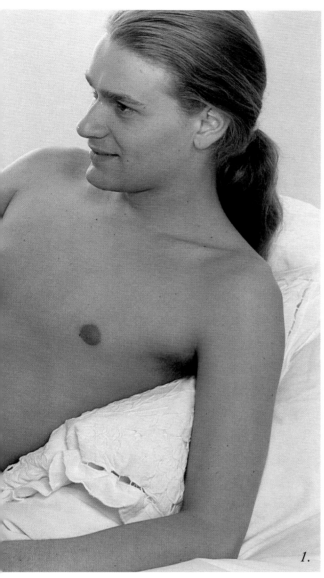

1.

While the best treatment for repetitive strain injury is rest and a variation in the offending habitual movement, massage is a good preventative method to help keep the hands relaxed and flexible.

When people think about giving a massage, they seldom consider a hand massage. In fact the hands, which do so much, are often one of the most neglected parts of the body. Yet even a short period of time spent massaging the hands can do so much to bring a deep sense of comfort and relaxation.

Holding your lover's hand conveys a universal message in the human language of touch. Without words, it is a way of expressing empathy, trust,

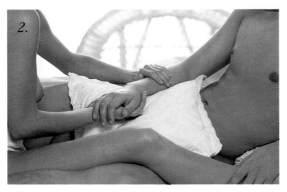

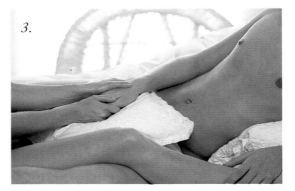

Mould your left hand into his wrist and arm and sweep it steadily up the forearm, encircling the elbow and gliding it lightly back down on the underside. Without pausing, pass his hand to your left hand, and use your right hand to repeat the movement on the inner side of his arm. Repeat these movements as a continuous sequence three times.

3. Now manipulate his hand to make space between those tiny bones and long tendons with circular strokes that simultaneously use the pressure from your heels to work the top of the hand and your

fingers to massage the palm. Support the palm with your fingers and, moving one hand after the other, work in circular movements from the knuckles to the wrist, increasing the pressure into your heels on the outer sweep of the circle. Glide back down and repeat the sequence three times.

4. Continue to support his hand with your fingers, but now use your thumb pads to make tiny circular movements, one thumb following the other, from the knuckles over the entire top of the hand and all around the wrist. This movement will take a little practice but is achieved by rotating the base joint of

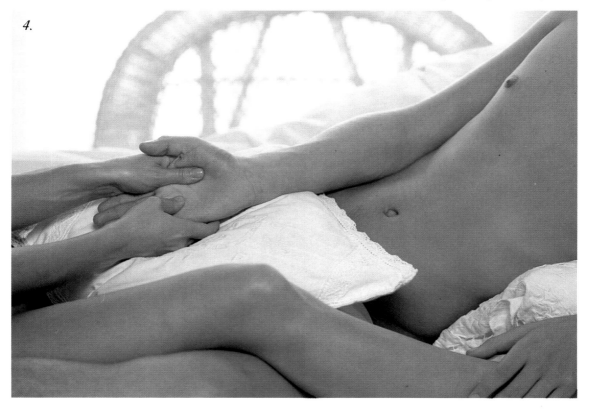

the thumb. Next, turn his hand over so the palm is facing upwards and repeat these thumb circles over its entire surface and up onto the wrist.

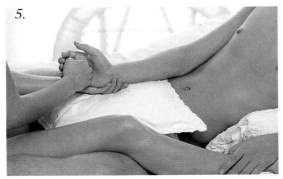

5.

5. Massage a little deeper into the palms by using your knuckles. Support your partner's hand with your left palm. Make a loose fist with your right hand and use the knuckles to make small semi-circular grinding motions over the entire palm.

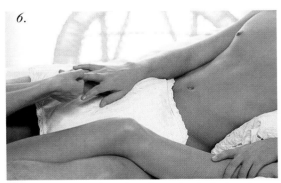

6.

6. Turn his hand so that the palm is facing downwards again. It is time to do the finger and thumb stretches that create the wonderful sense of tension being drawn right out of the body. Clasp the base of the little finger between the thumb and forefinger of your left hand and slide firmly but slowly along to its tip. Squeeze the end of the finger gently and snap out of its tip. Repeat these movements on the other fingers. Change to your right hand to pull along the forefinger and thumb.

7. Now sandwich your partner's hand between your own two hands and briskly rub back and forth to create an invigorating and heat-producing friction. Complete the massage by once more gently holding his hand between your own before repeating all the sequences on the left side. Spend a few moments in deep connection with each other, palm on palm.

TOUCH FOR STILLNESS AND CALM

Touching your loved one to soothe and relax him or her does not always involve massage strokes. The very nature of touch is that, with the right intent and a caring awareness, it provides a soothing and healing force. The 'laying of hands' on the body, as a means of calming, healing and removing pain or tension, is a natural and ancient practice as old as mankind itself. Unfortunately, these days we have all become so activity conscious and goal-orientated that we have almost forgotten the benefits of still-ness and silence and our own innate responses to the power of a loving touch. In the same way that we instinctively hold a painful area in our bodies, or a mother gently kisses away a 'nasty hurt' in her child, or a father's protective hand on the shoulder inspires confidence and trust, so we can extend that same simple hands-on gesture to our partners to bring them a feeling of relief and equilibrium.

This next programme is a series of simple holds accomplished by laying your hands in certain positions on and around your loved one's head and face. In doing so, you may be able to relieve tension headaches, or help empty an over-active mind. When you know your partner has been on mental overdrive, is anxious or just stressed-out, this simple head and face sequence can really help to let those worries dissolve. The beauty of this kind of motion-less hands-on work is that it can be as deeply relaxing for you to give it as it is for your partner to receive. It is very important for you to feel comfortable in your own posture, so if you are using your bed for the session, do ensure your back is well supported by cushions. You will want to create a peaceful atmosphere, so make sure you will not be interrupted. Keep checking that your own shoulders and wrists are relaxed, and take a few moments before you begin to breathe deeply into your abdomen. Continue this easy, slow breathing throughout the whole session, which lasts about 20 minutes. You do not need to use oil but your hands should be warm; by focusing your attention on them and being conscious of your breathing, you will be able to increase the natural body heat to this area. It is also important that you trust your hands and feel confident in their ability to create not only a physical release of tension but also an emotional

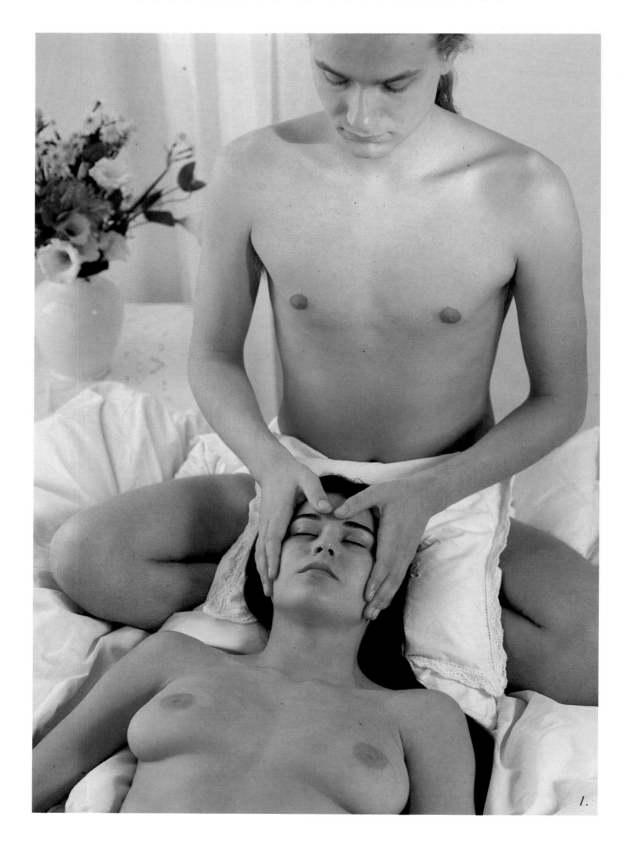

1.

support. Bring to your hands all your feelings of tenderness; let them be soft and supple; allow them to drop towards your partner's body with all the lightness of a silk scarf falling to the ground. Focus the heat and energy radiating from your palms on each area that you are aiming to relax but keep the whole of your hand supple and involved in the holds. Spend as long on each hold as you feel is necessary (which may be up to three minutes) and always draw your hands away slowly so that your partner hardly feels the break in contact.

A FACE AND HEAD SESSION

Sit, well supported, with your partner's head resting between your legs. If she has a lot of tension in the back of her neck, you may want to place a thin pillow under the base of her skull.

1. Begin by cupping your hands symmetrically over the sides of her face and temples, resting your thumbs alongside each other in the centre of her brow. When you are ready to withdraw, slide your hands up along the sides of her head so your thumbs glide up to her hairline. Run your fingers out through her hair.

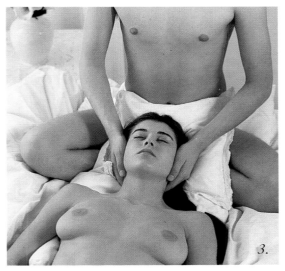

3. Cover her ears in the same soft and sensual way by cupping your hands over them. The heels of your hands should rest with very light pressure against her temples while your fingers point towards each other on the back of her neck. Release the hold by pulling your hands away very slowly.

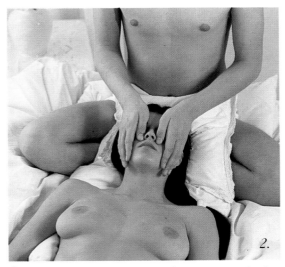

2. Bring the heat of your hands to warm and relax the tired, tense muscles that surround her eyes. Drop your hands confidently but lightly down onto her face so that the heels rest on her eyebrows and the palms softly cover her eyes. Your thumbs will lie just alongside her nose and your fingers will settle lightly over her cheeks and jaw.

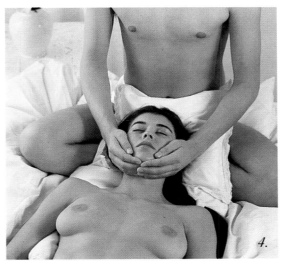

4. The jaw is often a key tension area and a tight jaw can increase stress throughout the whole body. Help those tensions melt with the warmth of your hands as they nestle each side of your partner's jawline, fingers meeting at her chin. When you are ready to complete this hold, lovingly slide your hands up over her jawline and out through her hair. Increase this relaxation by adding caressing strokes on each side of her jaw, one hand stroking after the other.

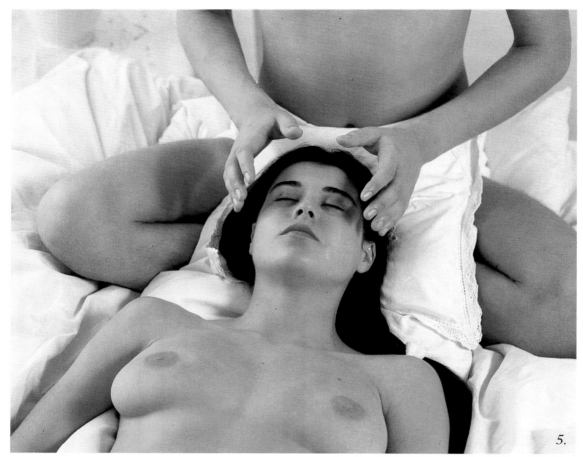

5.

5. Return your hands to cover the crown of your partner's head so that your fingers are pointing towards her ears and your thumbs are placed at the centre of the top of her forehead. Add a very slight pressure to your hands for a few moments and then gently release it. Continue to hold the symmetrical position of your hands as you draw them very slowly away from the head so your partner experiences this as a halo of heat expanding around her head.

6. Now cup the back of her head securely in your hands. To do this, gently roll her head into your left hand and slip your right hand under it. Roll her head to the right and place your left hand beneath it. Her head should be fully supported by your palms. Soften your hands so that they invite her head to drop its weight and melt back into them, thus allowing tension around her skull and the back of her neck to dissolve. When you are ready, gradually draw your hands from under her head so that it sinks slowly back to the mattress.

7. Help to release a stiff neck by sliding both hands under it so that your fingers are crossing over each other. As the heels of your hands rest on the edge of her skull, your palms will be generating a relaxing heat towards the muscles. After some time, pull your fingers steadily up the back of her neck and head, combing them out through her hair in soothing strokes.

8. By now your partner should be feeling very relaxed and able to let go of any mental strain accumulated during the day. Help her to integrate that sense of calm in her mind with the rest of her body. By placing your hands over the heart area you will also enable her to relax more into her feelings. Let your hands rest on her body so that the heels are just below the collarbone, the palms above the breasts and the fingers connecting to the centre of her chest. When you have completed this session, take time to lie together and relax. Let go into the beauty of simply 'being' together.

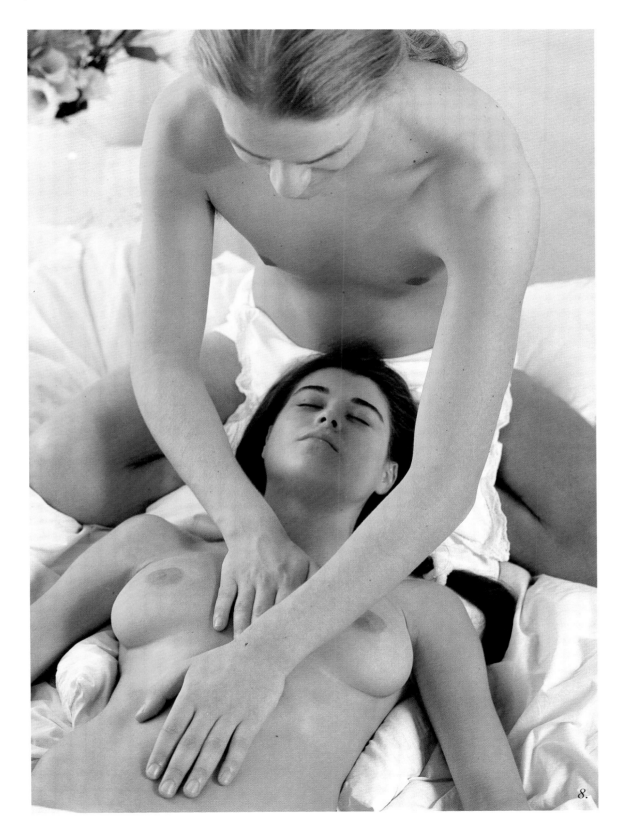

8.

Releasing
sexual tensions

In nature, all living organisms pulsate with vital energy because the movement

of life energy is like a wave – a constant cellular contraction and expansion.

In human beings, that vibrant motion of life-force is at its most apparent during

sexual orgasm when the whole body surrenders to involuntary and undulating

muscle movements and sensations of sheer pleasure.

YET FREQUENTLY, the capacity to yield fully to the joy of love-making is blocked by deep-rooted sexual tensions held within the body's musculature. These tensions act like armour within the the body so that it becomes stiff and ungiving, making it difficult to relax during love-making and to reach an orgasm. Even if orgasm occurs, it may be an unsatisfying feeling little more than a genital sneeze – a simple release from a localized build-up of sexual excitement.

While sexual tension manifests itself in the body's tissues, its origins are usually emotional. This is because our sexuality is not something that operates separately from our deepest thoughts, feelings and attitudes towards ourselves and others. Sexuality is a powerful primal energy and one that is often suppressed, consciously or unconsciously, whenever there is discomfort or judgement about the physical and emotional feelings related to it. Chronic tensions in the body, and particularly in the pelvic area, often have their roots in early childhood and adolescence. Children learn to control their emotions and intuitive responses and to hide their fears by restricting their breathing, especially exhalation, and by tensing their abdominal muscles.

The calm, still contact of your hands on your partner's body will encourage breath to deepen and tensions to dissolve.

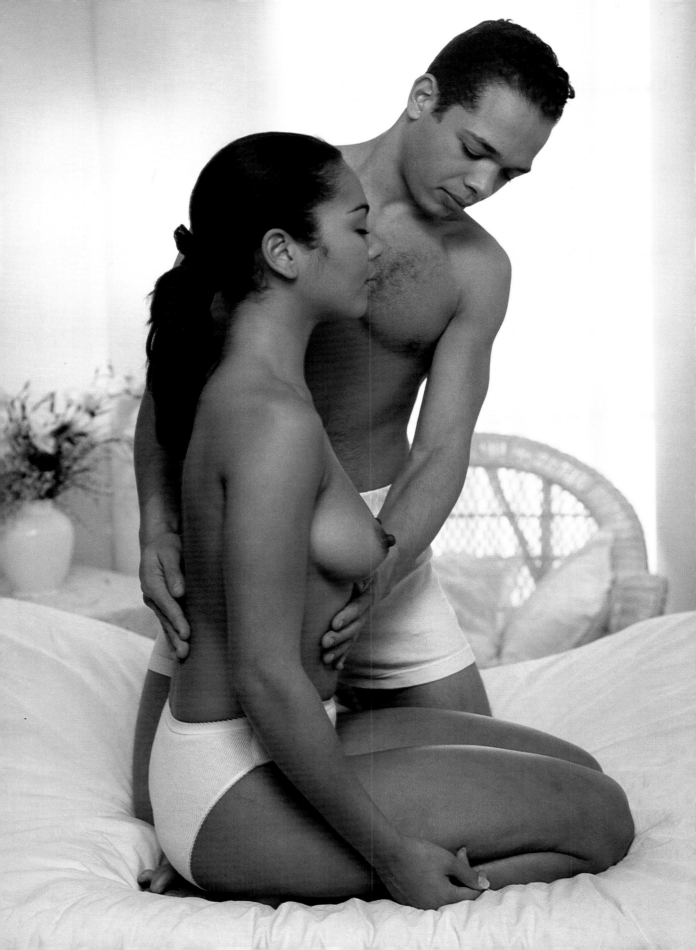

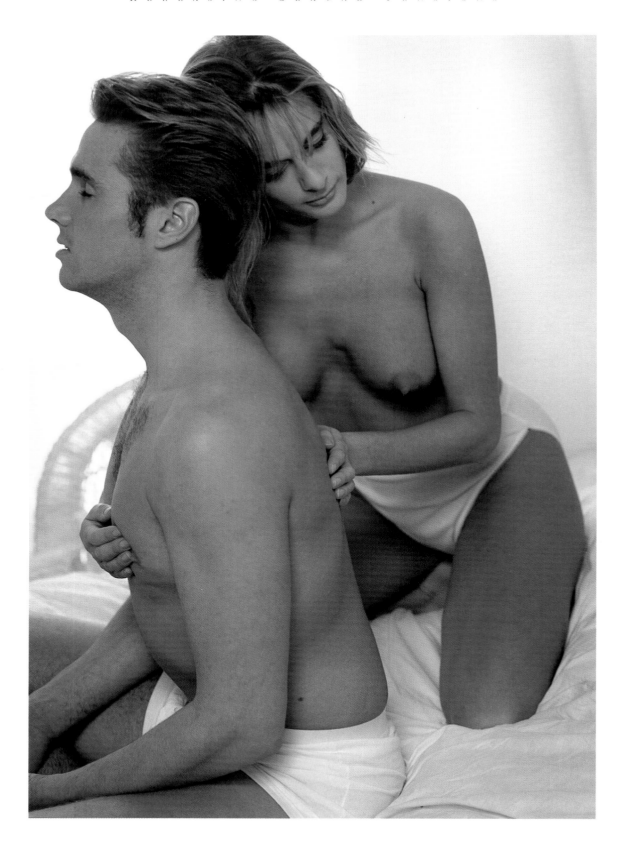

In so doing, they suppress 'gut-level' sensations such as anxiety, anger and pleasure. The reasons for inhibiting the natural responses of the belly and genital area can be numerous. Harsh toilet training, punishment for masturbation or for displaying emotions such as crying or rage, being told that 'down there is dirty', criticism of emerging sexuality, sexual and physical abuse, fear of one's own genitals and sexual impulses and so on are all reasons why a growing person will inhibit breathing and tighten muscles, thus cutting off spontaneous movement and feelings and natural sexual energy.

Over time, the now unconscious pattern of reduced breathing and muscular tension will affect physical and emotional spontaneity and 'aliveness'. This psychosomatic effect will manifest itself in many different ways in a person's life, and can certainly contribute to some degree of sexual dysfunction, anxiety or fear.

For example, the pelvis, which should be able to move freely during love-making, may feel rigid and unable to move separately from the whole trunk of the body, causing the person to force movements or feel like a block of wood. The abdomen, which could be pulsating with pleasurable sensations, may feel dead and unresponsive. Such tensions in the pelvic area, and the corresponding suppressed emotions, can lead to a number of sexual problems, including premature ejaculation or impotency in men and vaginismus, fear of penetration and inability to achieve orgasm in women. Sometimes, sexual tension can cause a 'split' between emotional intimacy and physical satisfaction and this can be damaging to a sexual partnership because one or both partners are unable to bring all aspects of themselves to a loving relationship.

Both men and women are affected by this level of sexual tension, though its manner may differ in either gender. For instance, a woman may complain that although her partner is technically a good lover, their love-making never feels intimate. She may

Vulnerable and tender feelings are often suppressed by tense musculature in the chest region. Help your partner to contact them by placing your hands gently over either side of the heart.

have achieved an orgasm but she does not feel cherished. She is puzzled as to why her man immediately withdraws from her emotionally the moment he has ejaculated. A man may not understand why his loving and caring partner is uninterested in sex, or derives little pleasure from it and remains unresponsive to his love-making.

Patience and understanding are needed by both partners if time is to be given to discovering and releasing the tensions and underlying feelings that are inhibiting their sexual enjoyment of each other. While some anxieties are so deeply embedded that professional counselling or psychotherapy are needed to enable traumatic memories and painful emotions to be unravelled and resolved in a neutral, safe and supportive way, there is much that two people in a trusting relationship can achieve through hands-on techniques to begin the process of relaxation. Not surprisingly, the body is often willing to release its tensions in response to supportive and loving touch.

It is important that if you are working on a sensitive issue such as the release of sexual tension your massage is not, at this point, goal-orientated towards making love; it is more an opportunity for your partner to experience body awareness, relaxation and release for its own sake. Any pressure towards, and expectation of, intercourse will only increase the tensions. In time, as both you and your partner experience the pleasure of getting to know these parts of the body, and accept and enjoy the sensations that come with deeper breathing, more mobility and relief from tension, your love-making is bound to become a richer experience.

RELAXING THE BELLY AND PELVIS

The belly and pelvis surrounds and supports the reproductive and sexual organs and is the part of the body most directly related to our sexuality. In the effort to repress gut-level feelings of sexuality, pleasure, anxiety or anger, muscles tighten across the abdomen and diaphragm and the exhalation of breath is reduced. Contracted muscles in the lower back, an extended belly and a retracted pelvis might also indicate a resistance to letting go into sexual impulses because of a negative belief about your sexuality.

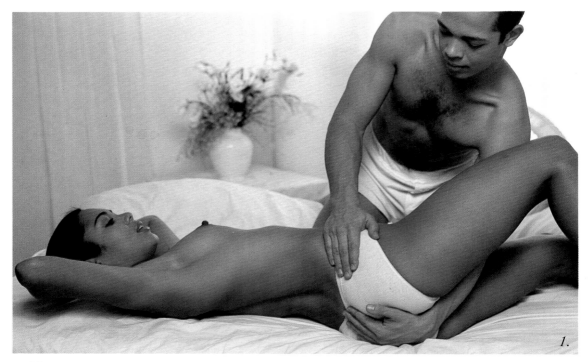

1.

To receive the belly and pelvis relaxation session, it is important to work only with someone whom you trust and who is able to respect your more vulnerable feelings. By increasing respiration into your belly and allowing the full release of exhalation, you may become aware of the muscular tensions and their underlying feelings. This body and breath awareness, together with the caring touch of your partner's hands on your skin, will encourage tight abdominal muscles to soften and tensions to dissolve. Emotions and sexual feelings may arise as vitality and relaxation in the area increases, but if you can trust and accept the rediscovered feelings, you will allow a natural and greater aliveness to infuse your body.

If you are giving this session, do remember that the belly is a very sensitive area beneath which lie important internal organs without the usual protection of bones. It is normal for anyone to jump away from sudden contact, so always approach the belly slowly and sensitively with your hands. The breathing should be a natural flow of inhalation and exhalation and never forced. If your partner's breathing is shallow or unfocused, you may want to verbally encourage her to breathe deeper by saying something like, 'As you inhale, imagine that you are sending your breath gently down into the area beneath my hand – now exhale as softly and as fully as you can', but make this sound like a subtle suggestion and not an order. If you use the wrong tone while telling your partner to relax or breathe more deeply you may create more tension or even resentment. You need to impart the feeling, both through your words and touch, that you completely accept your partner as she is right at this moment, and if any change happens it is always at her pace and choice. The very quality of this acceptance of the person as she is is one of the most healing aspects of massage and bodywork.

Always remember that tension originally forms in the body to protect a person from experiencing emotional or physical pain and it must always be respected. If you can just be there with your partner at the point of her tension, without pursuing a preconceived goal, you will create the all-important sense of safety and trust through which she can connect with and explore any pain, fears, emotions and anxieties which may be at the root of the tensions. A deep relaxation will come only when she is ready to release that tension of her own volition, but with your help to bring her conscious attention to her breath and body, she can begin the process.

BEGINNING THE RELAXATION

1. Start by kneeling beside your partner's left hip and ask her to roll her right hip towards you by raising her knee and using the pressure of her foot against the mattress. Wrap your right hand around the raised hip area and slide your left hand between her legs and beneath her buttocks to rest beneath the triangular flat bone of the sacrum at the base of her spine. Now ask her to roll back so her pelvis feels relaxed and the sacrum is nestled comfortably in the palm of your hand. At this point she should drop the right leg back down to the mattress and move around until she feels securely supported by your hand beneath her body.

2. Place your right hand (or hand nearest to her head) over your partner's abdomen just below the breastbone, and ask her to bring all her attention to the touch of your hand. She should now consciously direct her incoming breath into her abdomen so that your hand will feel the rise and fall of the belly with each inhalation and exhalation. Make your hand as receptive and sensitive as possible, allowing it to 'tune-in' to any subtle internal movement. This focus of inner and outer attention of breath and touch to the belly will begin the gentle release of tension as the muscles begin to expand and relax. As a result of releasing tension the belly may start making rumbling noises, but treat this as a positive sign of stress release and welcome it rather than getting embarrassed.

Spend between one and three minutes placing your hand on one area of the belly at a time. Once you feel it relaxing, place your hand on another part, including the area just above the pubic bone and then along the inner ridges of the pelvic girdle.

3. Once you have relaxed the whole abdomen in this way, complete the pelvic release by enabling the pelvic girdle to drop further towards the mattress. This is to bring a message of relaxation to the tense back muscles which cause the pelvis to retract. Raise the fingertips of your left hand so they indent slightly on the area just above the sacrum. Lean back with your body weight and draw this hand slowly out from beneath the sacrum and buttocks as if you were lengthening the base of the spine. Then slide your hand out from under the buttocks. This exercise is now complete, but you can relax the belly even more by giving it a gentle massage with oil. The additional strokes will warm and soften the abdominal muscles.

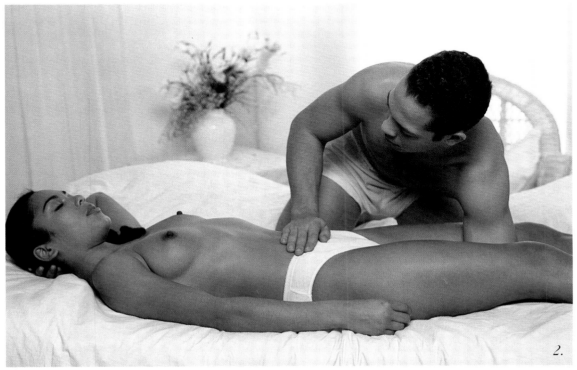

2.

BELLY MASSAGE

1. Rub a few drops of oil onto your palms and place your right hand on the top of the abdomen just below the breastbone and your left hand just above the pubic bone. Now slide the whole surface of your hands in smooth-flowing clockwise circular movements over the belly's circumference. The art of this stroke is to keep your left hand continuously moving in a complete circle, while your right hand only performs a half-circle stroke on the upper abdomen. Lift the right hand off the body to allow the top hand to pass beneath it and then return it to make another semi-circular movement. Massage the belly like this for up to five minutes, decreasing the circles to the centre of the belly and then expanding them out to the edges of the abdomen.

The body is three-dimensional, full of beautiful curves and contours which connect its back, sides and front and this rounded aspect of the pelvis and belly region can be conveyed to your partner by strokes which embrace all of those parts in flowing, sensual movements.

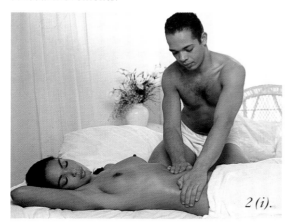

2 (i). Once you have massaged the surface of the belly with circle strokes, integrate it with the sides of the abdomen by a series of cross-over strokes to warm and relax the muscles which wrap across the sides of the body from the lower back to the belly. Put your left hand over your partner's right hip so that your fingers curl just beneath the back of her body. Place your right hand over her left hip so that your fingers rest lightly on the edge of her belly. Now glide both hands past each other over her belly to reach the opposite sides of her body and then back again to their original position.

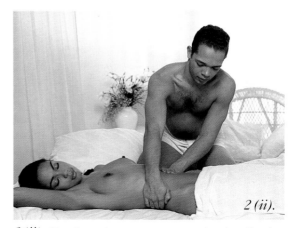

2 (ii). Continue these cross-over strokes in a flowing movement up over her abdomen and the sides of her body from her hips to her ribcage and back down again three times.

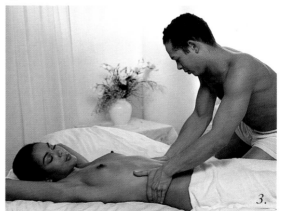

3. Now link the rounded shape of her hips and waist with her back by means of soft circular movements that fan up each side of her pelvis and abdomen. To do this, change your position so that you are still kneeling but are now facing your partner's head. Place your right hand over your partner's left hip and your left hand over her right hip. Sweep in small circular movements from her hips to her ribcage so that your palms caress the sides of her pelvis and abdomen while your fingers simultaneously stroke the back of her body. Draw your hands down along the back of her body, glide around her hips and repeat the sequence twice more.

4. Complete the massage with several more sweeping circular strokes over the surface of your partner's belly and then rest your hands softly over her abdomen for a few extra moments.

RELAXING THE THIGHS AND GROIN

At the height of the sexual act the strength and flexibility of the legs play an important part, not only in supporting the movements of the pelvis and the whole body and enabling exciting variations of love-making positions, but because the orgasmic discharge of energy from the genital area should be able to pulsate down through the legs and feet and out of the body. This is when the toes curl up in sheer ecstasy!

However, during love-making the legs can often feel tight, clumsy and unyielding, and even disconnected from the rest of the body. Both men and women hold tension in the inner and outer thigh muscles because of sexual anxieties about loosening up the genital and anal areas. This sequence of strokes and movements relaxes the legs by boosting the circulation and soothing the muscles to make them feel more alive and integrated with the whole body. Strokes on the thighs begin to warm and stimulate tight or flaccid muscles and precipitate a dissolving of tense holding patterns. The passive movements release contraction from around the hip joints and groin, creating a sense of spaciousness around the genitals.

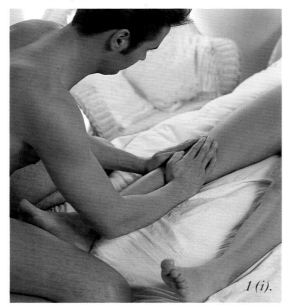

1 (i). Starting with your partner's right leg, stroke the oil down over her skin from her hip to her foot. Position yourself by her ankle and place both hands fully on her lower leg so that your fingers point towards her head. Firmly but gently, sweep both hands up the length of her leg, taking care to ease the pressure as you pass over her kneecap. As you reach her upper thigh, slide the hand closest carefully into the crease of her groin and let it rest on the top of the inside thigh. (Don't bump into the genital area as this will feel intrusive.) Glide your other hand on up to encircle the hip joint and pelvic girdle and back down the outer side of the thigh.

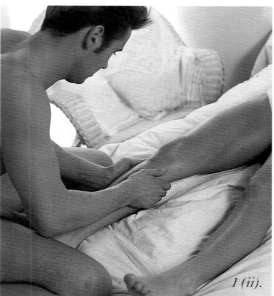

1 (ii).

1 (ii). When it is parallel with the waiting hand, draw both hands back down the leg with a firm, steady but relaxed stretch. Complete the stroke by pulling your hands out over the instep and sole of her foot, and repeat the whole movement up to five times without breaking the flow of motion.

2. Now kneel closer to her thigh so that you can focus your strokes on it. Let your hands be both pliable and strong, so that they mould into the shape of the thigh and yet move, stretch and revitalize the muscles beneath them.

Place your hands – fingers pointing towards your partner's head – on the centre of her thigh just above the knee. Stroke both hands upwards a short distance and then fan them outwards in opposite directions to encompass and glide back down the sides of her leg to where your strokes began. Return to the source of your stroke by flexing your wrists and gliding your hands lightly over her skin back to the centre of her thigh. This stroke will feel even better if you apply more pressure on the upward and outward movement of the fan motion, and glide back inwards more softly. Without breaking the continuity of the movement, repeat the full fanning movement but stroke up to a slightly higher position on her thigh. Fan stroke all the way up her thigh to the top of her leg and then slide your hands down the sides and back of her leg to just above her knee. Repeat the sequence twice more.

3. If your partner is holding sexual tension, she may be unconsciously protecting her genital area by tightening her inner thigh muscles. Adapt the circular strokes which you used to massage her belly to loosen and relax them. Gently open out her leg by letting it rest on your knee. Using both hands, stroke in circles up and down along the inside of her thigh from the groin to the knee until the muscles are rippling, loose and warm.

4. When tension is released from a certain area of the body during massage it is always beneficial to direct that release out of the body by the movement of your hands. After placing your partner's leg back flat on the mattress, stroke down the whole leg and out of the foot with your palms and fingers, one hand following the other in short overlapping movements.

5. Now position yourself comfortably so you can make the passive movements that lift the leg and open and relax the groin area. You will need to be

3.

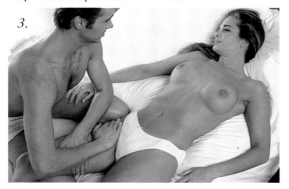

5.

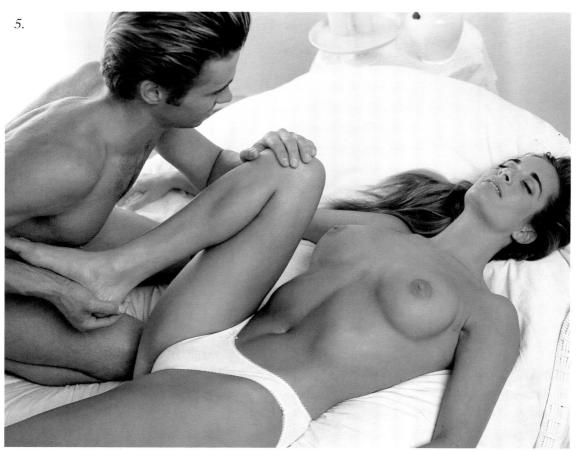

6.

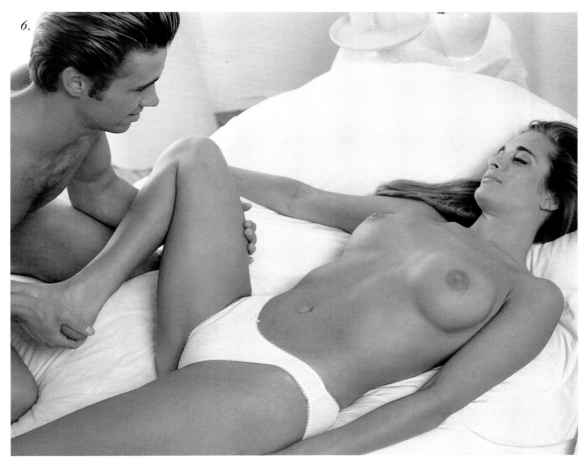

confident in your hands and steady in your own posture so that your partner feels able to trust you and relax the whole weight of her leg into your hands. The position of your hands will change depending on which leg you are moving. Start with her right leg, placing your right hand under her heel and your left hand under her knee to give it full support. Lever her leg upwards from the heel and as her knee flexes, slide your left hand over her knee and gently push it towards her body to create a slight stretch through her lower back, buttock and thigh. Ease her knee down towards her body as close as it can comfortably go without causing any strain. Ask your partner to breathe deeply into the releasing sensations of the stretch.

6. Slide your left hand to her outer thigh and allow the weight of her leg to fall against your hand. Lower her leg slowly outwards to create a sense of openness around her genitals and groin. Don't force the leg to open outwards beyond its point of tension or resistance – instead, encourage your partner into a deeper let-go by asking her to breathe down towards her genitals, and just rock her leg in tiny rhythmic movements on any point of tension you find. Chronic tension or holding does not disappear immediately, especially in such a highly charged sexual location as the groin. Be very patient and gentle and allow your partner to relax and open out her leg to the degree with which she feels comfortable.

7. Now bring her leg back in line with her body and, slipping your hand behind her knee to support it, lower her leg back down to the mattress. Repeat this whole sequence of strokes and passive movements on the other leg.

8. A lovely way to complete this session and to bring a feeling of calm and balance to her body is to place your hands over both feet and hold them for up to 30 seconds. The warm presence of your hands will bring a calmness to her whole body.

DISCOVERING THE ORGASM REFLEX

The term 'orgasm reflex' has been used by body-centred psychotherapists to describe the natural wave of involuntary movements that occur in the healthy body during sexual orgasm. Scientific research into this biological energy phenomenon was carried out thoroughly during the first half of this century by the controversial psychologist and medical doctor Wilhelm Reich. Reich, a contemporary of Freud, propounded the theory of 'character armour' – that is, that muscular tensions are formed within the body in direct relation to the suppression of emotions and natural sexual feelings. In doing so, Reich introduced the belief that by treating muscular tensions directly, and by helping patients release restricted breathing patterns, he could access the memories, traumas and patterns of repressive behaviour that led to neurosis and sexual dysfunction. By introducing physical contact and body techniques into his therapy to help free his patients from muscular tension and sexual repression, Reich alienated himself from the classic psychoanalytical movement and outraged conventional society.

Over the last half of this century, as acceptance has grown that the functions of body, mind and emotions are interlinked, the concept of treating the whole person has gained credence within the humanistic psychology movement and, increasingly, in the field of orthodox medicine and psychotherapy.

It is for this reason that massage, relaxation techniques and breath therapy are growing in popularity not only as a means to relax the body, but also to bring about psychological and emotional equilibrium.

Working with the orgasm reflex exercise can help you and your partner to become aware of the undulating movements that occur throughout the body naturally during orgasm but which are frequently restricted by muscular tensions. Since the whole body is involved in the orgasm reflex, start with a five-minute massage on the neck and head to unlock tight spots that may affect the wave of movement. Focus particularly on the area beneath the ridge of the skull to enable the head to move freely in response to the pelvic motion.

RELAXING THE HEAD AND NECK

1. Ask your partner to lie down on the mattress, taking time to relax her back against its surface. Rub just enough lotion or oil into your hands to lubricate your touch on her skin, as too much oil on the neck feels sticky and uncomfortable.

2. Slip both hands behind her neck so that your fingers are pointing downwards on each side of her spine. Allow your hands to become very soft and receptive so that her neck feels able to release tension and drop back towards your palms. Indent your fingertips slightly up into the muscle tissue and pull your hands confidently in a steady movement up her neck. Without breaking the movement, lift her head slightly as your hands pass the hairline so

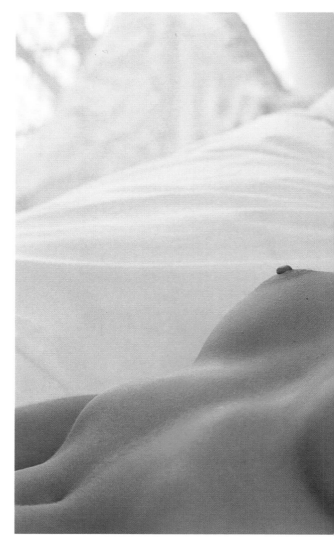

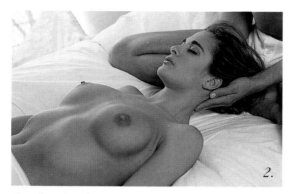

2.

that her head rests securely in your palms and continue to pull your hands out from behind her skull. Always take care not to pull her hair.

3. Using the fingertips of both hands, work smoothly in tiny continuous circular motions into the muscles at the back of her neck from its base to the skull line.

4. With her head now resting securely in the palms of your hands, press your fingertips up so they sink gently and slowly into the tissue immediately below the base of the skull. This area can be extremely tense, so apply pressure very sensitively. Allow her head to sink back into your hands while you maintain the pressure for about 30 seconds. You should now slowly release the pressure from your fingertips while lifting her head slightly upwards to give the neck a stretch. Lift her head in a straight line with the spine and encourage your partner to give its whole weight into your hands. Lower her head very slowly back down to the mattress.

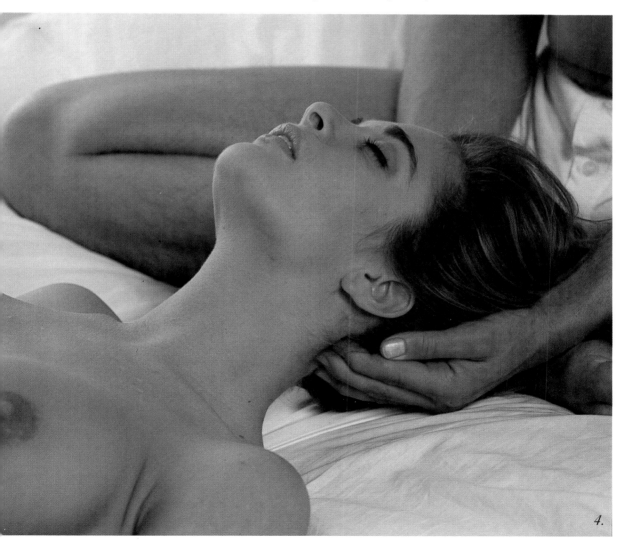

4.

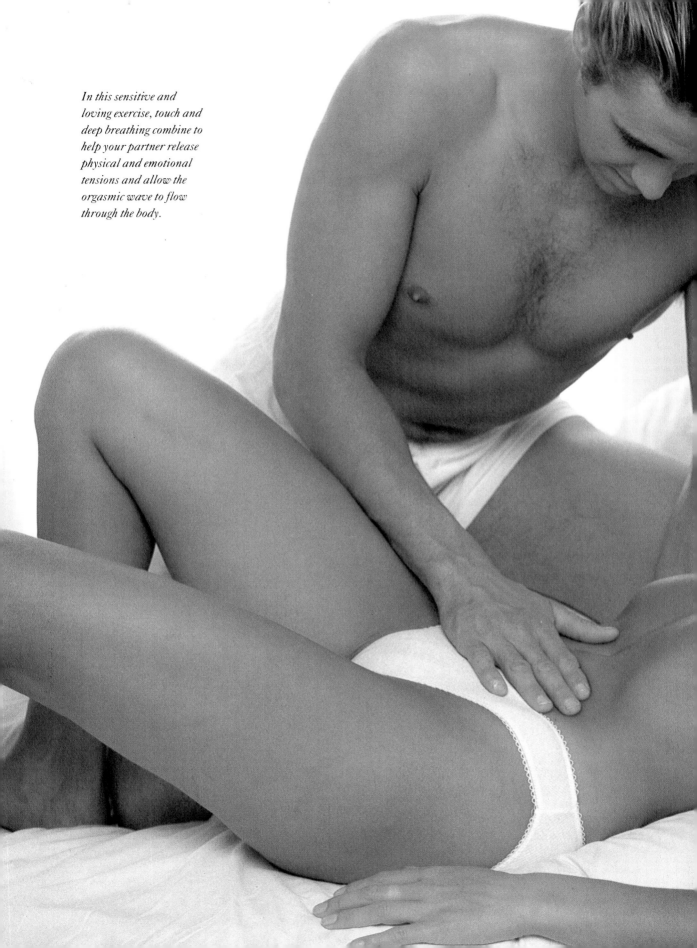

In this sensitive and loving exercise, touch and deep breathing combine to help your partner release physical and emotional tensions and allow the orgasmic wave to flow through the body.

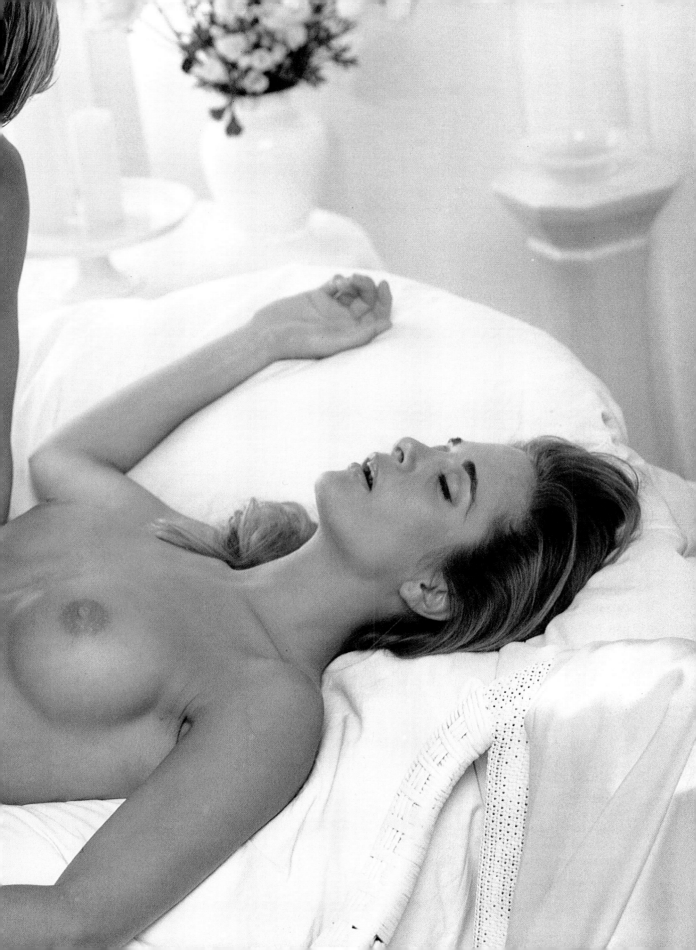

CREATING THE ORGASMIC WAVE

Spend up to 15 minutes on this exercise or for as long as your partner feels comfortable. As tension releases, she may experience sensations of heat and cold or even some vibration and shaking. It is possible that she may feel emotional and it is important to allow her to express what she is feeling if she wishes to do so. She may also feel a warm sense of aliveness in the lower abdomen, genitals and thighs and this tingling vibrant feeling will then flow easily throughout her entire body. Allow your partner to express these sensations in any way she feels and be sensitive to her responses.

1. Move your position to kneel beside your partner's belly. Ask her to support the weight of her legs by placing her feet firmly on the mattress about shoulder-width apart so that her knees are raised. Place one hand over her upper abdomen and the other below the small of her back. Encourage your partner to ease her back towards your hand so she can drop the tension in the pelvic girdle.

2. Ask your partner to breathe fully into the abdomen in the same manner as during the pelvic and belly release. As she inhales, her belly should extend slightly. On exhalation, the belly will relax and the pelvis and genital area should lift slightly up and forward, causing her legs and groin to open outwards naturally. At the same time, her head should tilt back and her shoulders move forward. This subtle wave of movement, combined with a deepening flow of breath, will begin to create a natural wave of energy throughout the body similar to the uninhibited orgasm reflex. Ask your partner to consciously encourage this motion within her body, but not to force anything.

3. As your partner's breathing deepens, depress your hand gently on her upper abdomen with the outflowing breath and lighten your touch with the inhalation. Your touch and her breath will help the diaphragm muscle to release its tension, letting go of constriction between the upper and lower parts of her body so that vital energy can stream through unimpeded. At some point, move your hand to the lower half of her belly (just above the pelvic bone) to encourage the breathing to reach into the pelvic floor and genital area. This will infuse the tissues surrounding her sexual organs with energy.

SEXUAL TENSION IN THE BUTTOCKS

The buttocks are a reservoir of sexual sensation, but tensions in their large, strong muscles can inhibit a fully sensual experience. Deep massage on the buttocks can release emotional and physical tensions and bring feelings of great relief and pleasure, as well as an easing of muscular aches and stresses in the lower back.

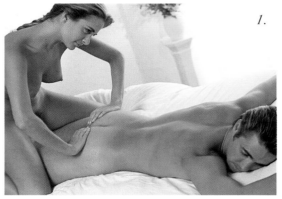

1.

1. Straddle the back of your partner's knees, taking care not to lean your weight on his body. Rub some oil between your hands and spread it over his thighs and buttocks with smooth, sensual strokes. This is a wonderfully curved part of the body, so let your hands slide and mould over its rounded contours. Slide your hands confidently yet sensitively over the back of his thighs so that your fingers stroke along his inner thighs and into the creases of his buttocks, then fan your hands symmetrically outwards over the pelvic girdle. Draw them back down over his hips and outer thighs and then repeat the stroke at least five times in a continuous flowing motion until the thighs and buttock muscles feel warm and relaxed.

2. Begin to massage deeper into the large buttock muscles to loosen tension. Increase the pressure into the heels of both hands and make continuous circular movements all over the fleshy area. Massage thoroughly into the crease between the buttocks and the top of the thighs. While making these circular strokes, remember to increase the pressure on the outward half of the circle and return more lightly. Once you have worked over the area thoroughly, soothe the skin and muscle tissue with soft strokes from the flat of your hands to accentuate the curvaceous lines of the body.

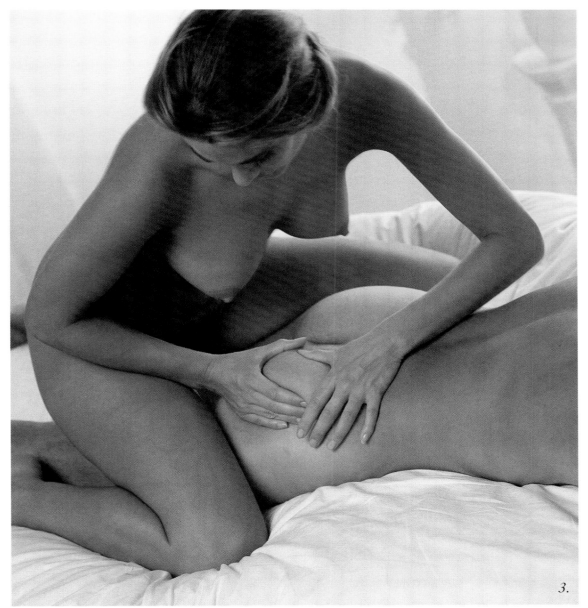

3.

3. Kneading strokes will invigorate the muscles and loosen a deeper level of tissue tension. These strokes feel very pleasurable and enlivening on fleshy areas such as the buttocks and thighs. Kneading is done by scooping and squeezing the flesh between the sides of the thumb and fingers of one hand and then rolling it towards the other hand. In a continuous back-and-forth motion between both hands, repeat the lifting, squeezing and rolling of flesh over the entire area of your partner's buttocks.

4. Again, soothe the buttocks with soft rounded strokes after the kneading. To complete the massage, stimulate the skin surface by making short downward and overlapping raking movements with the fingertips of both hands. Rake from the pelvic girdle, over one side of the buttocks and onto the thigh and then repeat on the other side.

5. Using a motion similar to raking, but with softer pressure, feather stroke the buttocks with your fingertips. Complete the massage by resting your hands softly over the buttocks for some moments.

Aqua-pleasure in massage

Our evolutionary origins were oceanic and to this day our bodies consist of 90 per cent salt water. Maybe this is the reason why the liquid caress of water on our skin helps us to relax and let go of tensions easily. In water we feel good about ourselves and our nakedness, returning to an almost child-like pleasure in our bodies.

THE RIPPLES OF water gently massage us and soften our muscles, their droplets running in tiny rivulets over the skin. The sensation helps to release us from everyday stresses and calls us back to a memory of nature and freedom: the sound of ocean waves, the cascade of a waterfall, the slow, lazy meandering of a river, the gentle patter of rain. Water is as sensual as it is therapeutic for body and mind, its fluidity embracing all material matter. At home, in the privacy of a bath or shower, we stretch and move our bodies, unselfconscious in our nakedness. We can lift our faces to welcome the watery spray while we touch and stroke ourselves intimately. Warm water will soothe aching muscles, and cold water will stimulate our circulation. As we rub our skin with soap, we massage ourselves. Water cleanses us internally as well as externally as we let it wash away our worries and refresh our minds.

Water brings pleasure. What then could be more natural than to use the setting of a bath or shower to explore and enjoy our own bodies, or to share the occasion with a partner in an exchange of tender touch? The following sequences of massage in a shower setting will add to your spontaneity of touch to turn an everyday event into something that is truly special.

Under the luxurious caress of warm water, nakedness and physical intimacy become spontaneous and uninhibited.

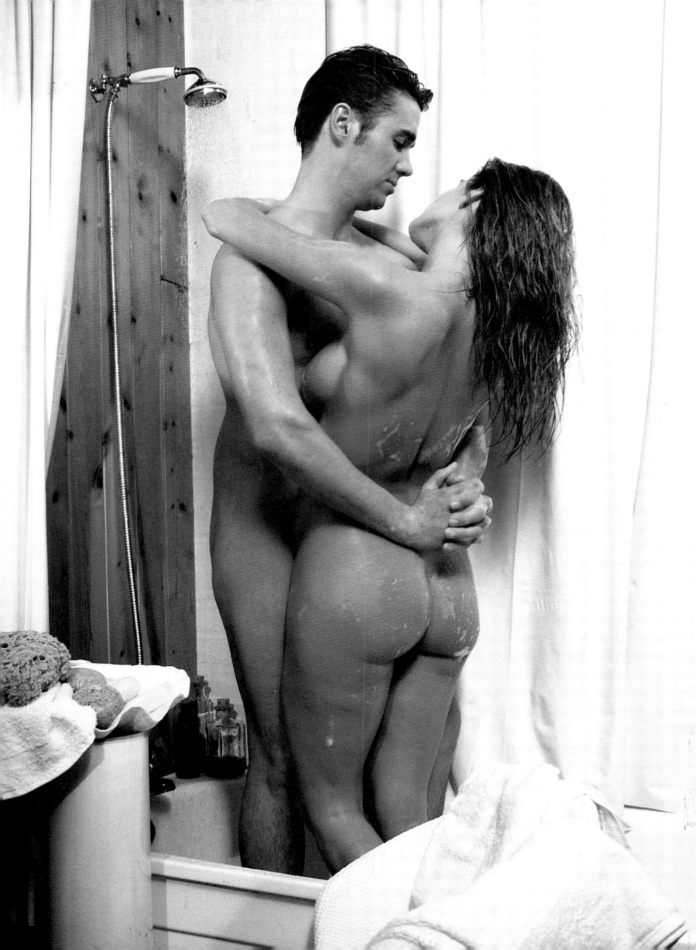

SELF-MASSAGE IN THE SHOWER

Learning to know and love our own bodies is an important step in the art of touching, massaging and making love. If we have a poor body image of ourselves, we carry these inhibitions and conflicts into the most intimate interactions with our partners. We cut off our spontaneity and instinctive responses. This is especially true for women, who frequently harbour negative thoughts about their body image – often without rational foundation. In fact, one magazine survey which sought to discover what rated as the most unappealing habit between

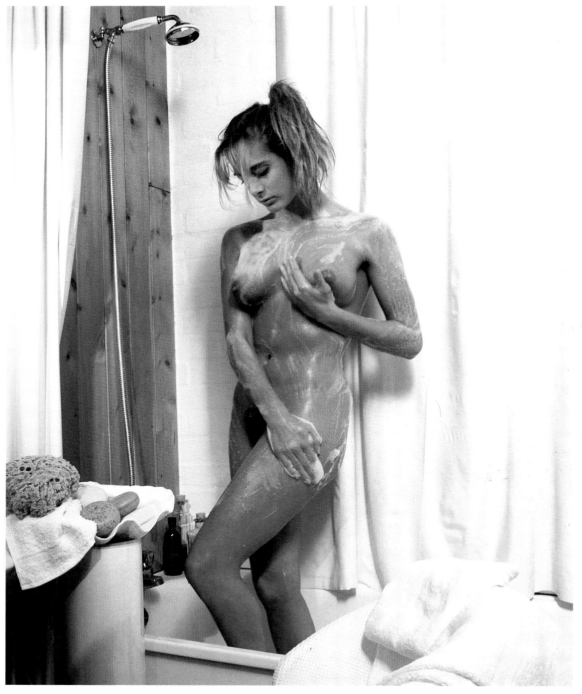

sexual partners found that women's critical judgements about their own bodies was high on the list of men's complaints. These negative and often unfounded beliefs made the men feel uncomfortable and embarrassed about their own bodies.

A good self-image arises not only from a sense of satisfaction with our external appearance, but also from a more intimate relationship with our bodies, feelings and senses. Showering naked provides a private opportunity for learning how to appreciate your own body without inhibition and how to touch yourself with wonder and tenderness. For self-massage in the shower, choose a time when you do not need to hurry. If it is evening, use candlelight in your bathroom to create a mellow and sensuous mood. Select soaps or gels that will nourish your skin. Then, as the gentle cascade of water brushes and stimulates your skin, discover how good your own touch feels when applied to your body with a loving sensitivity and awareness. Let your hands stroke and wander over every inch of soft, wet skin and slide with the lather of soap over every contour, crevice and curve. In the shower, there is no formal way to give yourself a massage – just play with your strokes and discover what feels good. Learn to let go of the tension in your hands so that they become soft and pliable, melting into your body shape with every caress. Encourage the strength and dexterity of your hands as they knead the fleshy parts of your body – the upper arms, thighs, sides of the hips and waist – and, at the same time, invigorate and relax tired, tense muscles. Tone up slack muscles on your arms and thighs and boost the blood circulation to the surface of your skin with quick vibratory percussion movements. There is no better way to start loving your own body while at the same time discovering what strokes will delight your partner.

Here are some suggestions to turn your everyday shower routine into a sumptuous occasion of self-appreciation and body care.

Learn the art of touch and how to appreciate your own body while you are taking a shower. Let your hands mould and slide over every contour as the warm water gushes over your body.

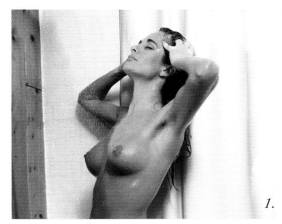

1.

THE HEAD AND FACE

1. While shampooing your hair, use tiny circular movements with the fingertips of both hands to massage thoroughly over your entire scalp.

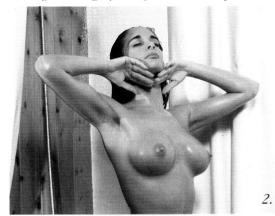

2.

2. Trace the delicate bone structure of your face with firm but gentle strokes. Use the fingertips of both hands to glide outwards from an imaginary central line running down your face. Start with your forehead, ending each movement with a sweep around your temples. Then stroke outwards under your eyebrows and below your eye-socket. Press the first two fingers of both hands on each side of the bridge of the nose and slide them down along the nose and out over the cheekbones. Rotate your fingertips in small outward flowing movements over the fleshy area of the cheeks. Then stroke the back of your fingers from the centre of the chin, up over each side of the jaw to the ears. Support the back of your ears with your thumb pads, and use the tips of both index fingers to massage in little circles all over the ears.

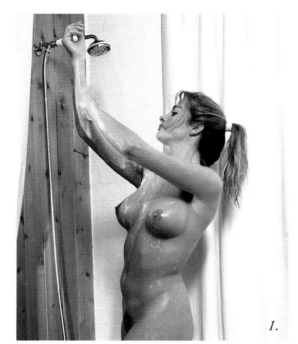

1.

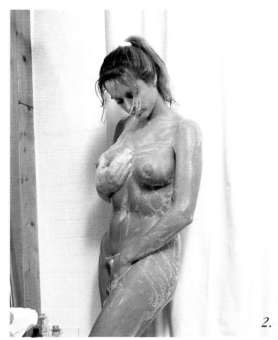

2.

THE ARMS

1. We use our arms to express so many sweet feelings in a relationship, embracing and enfolding a lover to our bosom, yet we seldom pay attention to them. Use your shower time to explore their shape and texture with your hands. Raise your face and chest up towards the fall of water and, lifting your arms, explore their wonderful range of movement. Play with the flexibility of your elbow, wrist and finger joints, and rotate your arms to loosen up the shoulder joints. Then, using one hand at a time, smoothly spread the lather down each arm from the fingertips to the shoulder and watch how little streams of soapy water snake their way sensuously down onto your body.

TORSO AND LEGS

2. Think of your body as a gently undulating landscape to be explored by soft strokes and lingering caresses with your hands and fingers. Touch yourself as you would like to be touched by your lover. Let the flat surface of your hands slip and slither over the rounded formations of your various body parts, integrating the different areas with long sweeping strokes. Moulding your hands to your body shape, glide them over your buttocks and hips, waist and belly, chest and ribcage. If you are a woman, cup your breasts in your hands and gently palpate them, then slide your hands around and around their circumference. Caress your belly, one hand following the other in clockwise motions. Follow the full, sensuous shape of your buttocks with rounded motions and then slip your hands over the front of your legs to the soft skin of your inner thighs. Stroke delicately with your fingers up over your genitals, then move your hands over your belly and chest and on up to your shoulders in long, sweeping strokes. Lean forward to circle your hands down each leg from thigh to ankle, returning them with an upward sweep over the back of the leg.

TIPS FOR INVIGORATING STROKES

• Make a loose fist with one hand and pummel across the top of the opposite shoulder, flicking your fist off the skin as soon as it makes contact.
• Use one hand to knead down the fleshy area of the opposite arm with a lifting, squeezing and releasing motion.
• Stimulate the circulation and tone your hips and thighs with a quick hacking motion. Keep your wrists loose and use the sides of both hands alternately to quickly strike the skin in rapid and rhythmic succession. Alternately, you can pummel your thighs to help eliminate cellulite.

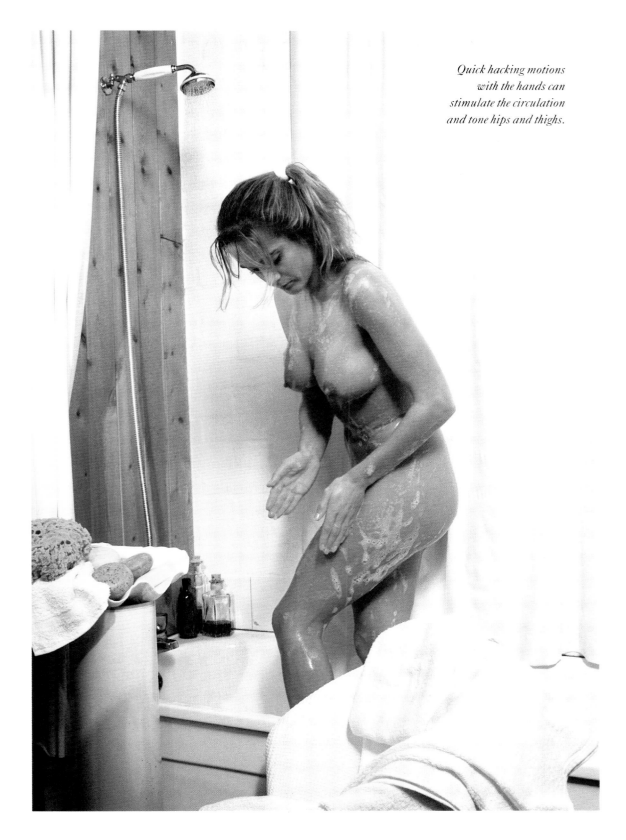

*Quick hacking motions
with the hands can
stimulate the circulation
and tone hips and thighs.*

SHOWERING WITH YOUR PARTNER

Water is a nurturing presence from the earliest moments of our lives. During the nine months in the womb, a foetus floats in a soft cushion of amniotic fluid that protects it from internal and external pressures and shocks. Later on, the bathtime ritual provides a small child with an opportunity to play with and relate to its own body. Splashing around in the water, the naked baby learns about its body in the best possible way – through loving touch from its parents without shame or embarrassment.

It is so natural to be without clothes in the shower that bathing with your lover, and combining the experience with massage, can re-create that childlike sense of wonder and innocence in the exploration of the body. It is an occasion to cherish each other and, at the same time, celebrate your sensuality.

Showering together, you can take it in turns to massage weary shoulders, neck and arms, and ease away tensions with a scalp massage while washing each other's hair. You can make the occasion as sensuous as you wish. Let your hands free-flow all over your partner's body as you soap the wet skin. While you spread the lather, let your hands be as fluid in movement as the water that has washed over both of your bodies.

Gently and tenderly, let your hands wander and explore each other's nakedness. Your bodies can move and slide together easily with the slipperiness of the soap in an all-body mutual massage. On a practical note – with all that movement and lather happening in your shower, it is probably a good idea to use a slip mat!

Be as spontaneous and instinctive as you feel while showering with your partner. There is no set format to follow with your water massage, but here are some suggestions that will enhance it.

A BACK MASSAGE

The anatomy of the human back, with its wonderful lines and contours, has always been celebrated in classic art forms, yet we know little about the physical appearance of our own backs. Also, unless we are adventurous while making love, the back may remain mostly unseen and untouched during intimate moments. So use the opportunity of showering together to make real physical contact with the back. Through your hands, you can reveal to your partner the shape of his back and the length of his spine, the tapering in of his waist and the angles of his hips. While stroking his upper back, you can trace the triangular formation of his shoulder blades and the slope of his shoulders. By easing away tension from his back, you will help both his body and mind to relax.

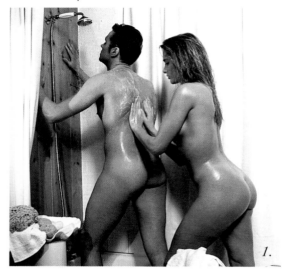

1.

1. Begin with a flowing main movement over the whole of his back. Place the flat of your hands, fingers pointing towards his head, on either side of his lower spine. Slide your hands steadily upwards over the long muscles that support the spine, moulding them out and over the shoulders and top of the arms. Pull your hands firmly down the sides of his body so that they sculpt his ribcage and waist and fan out and around his hips. Flex your wrists so that your hands glide back to their first position and repeat the whole movement four times.

2. To relax his upper back and shoulders adapt the strokes used in Massage for Easing Shoulder and Neck Tension (page 18). By kneading and massaging the shoulders you will decrease stress.

3. Placing your hands over each hip, stroke them up the sides of his body in spiralling circles to the edge of his shoulder blades. Curve your hands in towards the centre of his back and out again down to his hips. Repeat the sequence twice more.

4. Fan stroke up from the base of his back to the top of his shoulders. Place both hands, fingers pointing

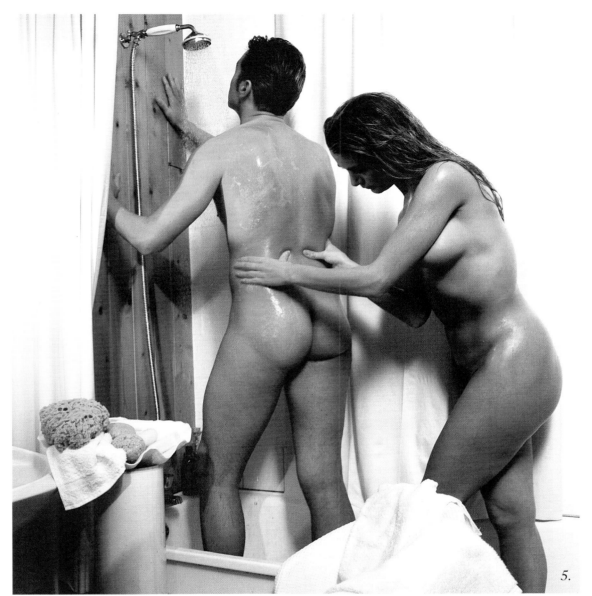

5.

towards his head, flat on each side of his spine. Push them about 15cm/6 inches up his back before spreading them outwards like an open fan. Let your fingers embrace and stroke back down the sides of his body before flexing your wrists and gliding your hands lightly back to a position just above where your last stroke began. Repeat the motion all the way up his back to his shoulders, expanding the fanning movement to cover the broad surface of the top of his back. Now draw your hands sensuously down the ribcage and back to where you began your strokes. Repeat the sequence twice.

5.   Massage a little deeper alongside his spine. Place both thumb pads beside the vertebrae of the lower back. Lean your body weight into your thumbs, but keep your hands softly on his back to support your strokes. Massage up along the edges of the vertebrae with both thumbs simultaneously, rotating in tiny circles, until you reach his shoulder blades. These pressure strokes will ease away strain along the spine. Fan your hands up and over his shoulders and back down the sides of his body. Circle them around his hips to a position where they can repeat the sequence once more.

MELTING FRONT TO FRONT

An even more sensual way to massage the back is to face your partner so that you have full frontal body contact. Place your arms around each other, so that your bodies merge and melt.

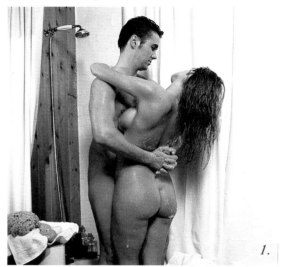

1.

1. Interlink your fingers, and by moving your wrists and applying pressure to the heels of your hands, rotate the edge of the heels up alongside her spine from the small of her back to her shoulder blades and back down again.

2. Keeping the same intimate position, use the wide surface of the underside of both forearms to create alternate and sweeping circular movements over the whole of her back.

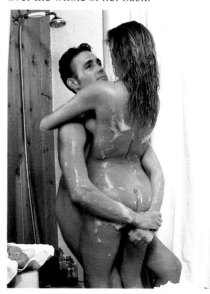

3 (i).

3 (i). Now get ready for a wonderful buttocks lift and spinal stretch (this stroke can only work if the active partner is taller than the receptive one). Have your partner raise her arms so that her hands are linked together behind your neck. Bend your knees so that you are low enough to wrap your arms around her just below her buttocks. To secure your hold of her body, use one hand to grip the wrist of your other arm. Using a hugging motion, slide firmly up over her buttocks with your forearms so that the whole area is lifted upwards.

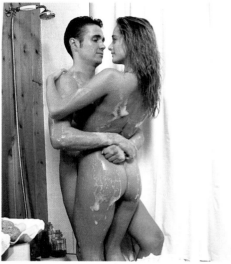

3 (ii).

3 (ii). Continue to pull your arms steadily up over her back and spine with this lifting motion until you are standing straight.

WASHING THE GENITAL AREA

The buttocks, belly, thighs and genitals form the intimate part of the body. The naturalness of your mutual nudity in the shower will remove any awkwardness in lovingly washing, massaging and caressing this area. To reach this part of the body easily, kneel with one foot on the ground for support. From this position you can massage both the back and front of the body without difficulty.

1. Softly define the full rounded shape of his buttocks with flowing strokes from both hands. As they encircle his hips, let your fingers deftly stroke over the front of his pelvis.

2. Massage and relax the inner thigh muscles. Use the underside of your forearm to massage in circles on the inner leg from the knee towards the groin.

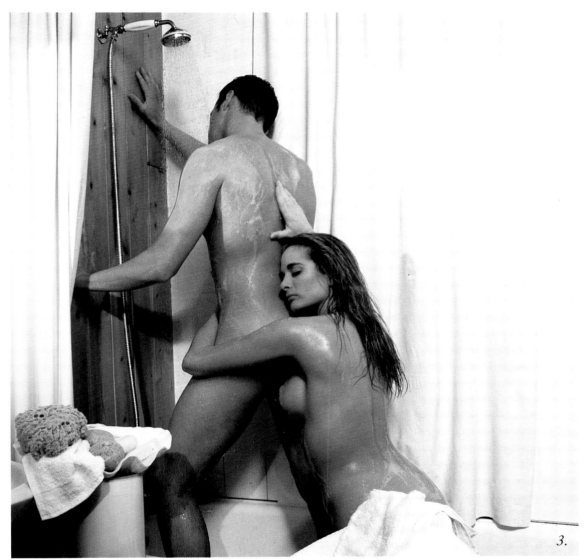

3.

3. Rest your head gently against the curve of the lower back and wrap your arms around his hips so that you can wash and stroke his belly and genital organs. With one hand following the other, sensitively caress his scrotum and penis.

MASSAGING THE CHEST, BREASTS AND BELLY

A woman's breasts are highly sexually sensitive, yet most women resent having their breasts demarcated specifically as a sexual zone. In this tender and sensuous shower massage, let your hands appreciate the whole beauty of her body as they flow over her chest and belly and embrace her breasts.

1. Stand so that you can support your partner as she leans her upper body against your chest. Try to merge in to each other's rhythm of breathing, letting it be deep and relaxed.

2. Place both your hands lightly over the soft roundedness of her belly so that your fingers are pointing down towards her pubic bone. Slide your hands gently up over her belly and then fan them smoothly out and down over each side of her abdomen until your fingers meet. Now swivel your hands back to their original position and repeat the stroke several times in a constant motion. This wonderfully fluid movement will relax and warm her belly.

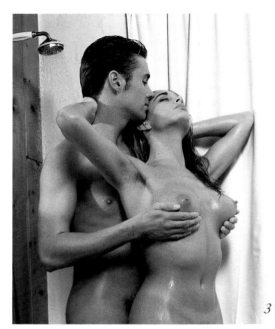

3

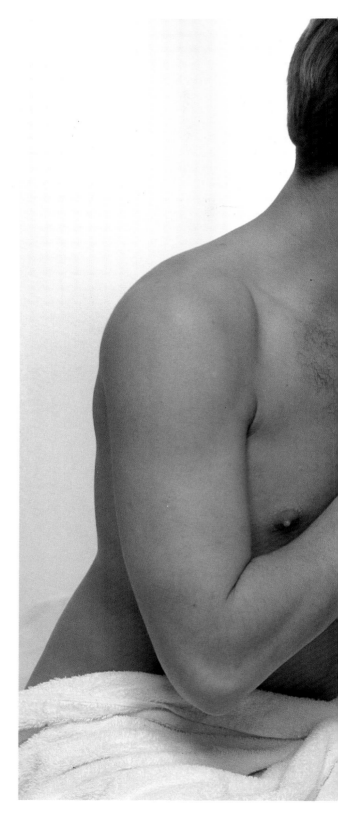

3. Slide your hands up over her belly and then, one hand following the other, stroke along the length of her breastbone. Pull your hands out over each side of the pectorals – the muscles above the breasts – in a movement that brings a feeling of expansion to the upper chest. Without breaking the flow of your stroke, flex your wrists so that your hands can glide along the sides and directly beneath her breasts and back up her breastbone. Encircle her breasts in this way several times. Then gently cup her breasts in your hands, and hold them lovingly in a still and sensitive way.

AFTER THE SHOWER

When your shower is complete, continue to cherish each other. Wrap your partner snugly in a warm, clean bath towel and pat over the whole body to dry it. Gently towel dry the hair. Now anoint and moisturize one another's skin with oils or lotions. Relaxed and open to one another, you are ready for an occasion of sensual delight.

After bathing together, your bodies will feel particularly warm and supple and the skin soft and vibrant.
The intimate mood created by shower massage can be enhanced by rubbing oils and lotions onto the body to nourish the skin.

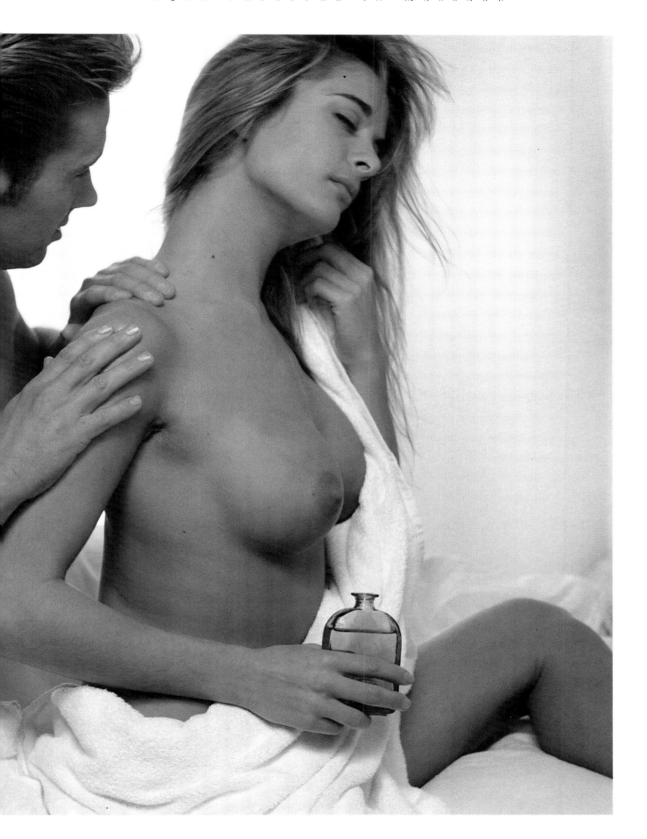

A FOOT BATHING RITUAL

In many traditional societies, the bathing and anointing of another person's feet are acts of hospitality offered as a matter of course to a welcomed guest. In Eastern cultures, such as that of India, people commonly touch the feet of an elder, parent, teacher, friend or guest as a sign of deep respect. It is perhaps difficult for the Western mind to understand that such a gesture is born out of a sense of honour and devotion and does not signify inequality or servitude.

In Western cultures, there is more of a taboo about the exposure and touching of feet than any other part of the body except the genitals and breasts. People are very coy about their feet, and rarely expose them, except on a beach or beside a pool. Feet are usually hidden away, huddled in uncomfortable shoes and socks so that they become cramped and almost lifeless. Unlike the rest of the body, they are rarely pampered, and even the best dressed and manicured people may be embarrassed if they have to expose their unloved feet. Perhaps that is the reason why the tabloid press and public are so fascinated with the 'toe-sucking' exploits of the rich and famous!

Yet we should learn from the East, because few things can convey appreciation and love for someone as much as the touching and massaging of feet. Combined with a specially prepared foot bath, infused and steaming with healing aromatic oils or herbs, or a simple cleansing natural salt bath, a feet treat will take the weariness out of tired, aching legs and feet, restore and relax the entire body and revive the spirit.

So spoil your partner with a foot massage and foot bath. Prepare the setting carefully to make the event a special occasion. Heat the room to a comfortable temperature and turn on soft lighting. You will need a foot bowl that is big enough for both feet to spread out and soak in ankle-deep water, together with warm towels to pat dry the legs and feet. Use a chair in which your partner can easily relax and a cushion or low footstool where you can sit by her feet to give the massage.

Begin by preparing a footbath of warm water to which you add your essential oils or sea salt. Then perform the massage on the lower legs and the feet.

AROMATIC FOOT BATH

Carefully select the essential oils to evoke the specific mood and effect you wish to create. Aromatic oils, which are usually available in health and beauty shops, are extracted from plants, flowers and herbs and contain remedial properties which beneficially effect both body and emotions. They are very potent, and only a few prescribed drops should to be used in the bowl of water. Here are two recipes, one to soothe and relax, the other to restore and invigorate. Each contains five drops of a mixture of suitable essential oils.

Footbath to relax:	Footbath to invigorate:
2 drops of lavender	*1 drop of teatree*
2 drops of bergamot	*2 drops of geranium*
1 drop of camomile	*2 drops of orange*

A SIMPLE CLEANSING FOOTBATH

Throw a small handful of natural sea salt into a bowl of warm water and stir until the granules have dissolved. Sea salt is known to be a natural cleansing agent, drawing the body's toxins out of the skin and relaxing the tissues. It is also rich in minerals.

Once you have prepared the bowl of warm water and added to it your chosen ingredients, place it before your partner, and ask her to soak her bare feet for five minutes. Suggest that she flexes and stretches her toes and feet in the water to exercise the tendons and muscles and release tensions. You will probably hear her sigh with relief as her feet begin to relax.

THE FOOT MASSAGE

A foot massage benefits the whole body. The foot has many thousands of nerve endings which are stimulated during a massage. There is even a whole system of pressure-point therapy practised on the feet, called reflexology, which works by pressing with thumbs or fingertips on specific zones to boost corresponding organs, glands and body areas. Each foot contains 28 small bones and long tendons running down from the leg muscles to the toes.

1. Take her right foot out of the bowl and enfold it with a warm towel. Gently pat her foot to dry it thoroughly and place it on your knee. Make sure your partner's leg is relaxed and the knee flexed.

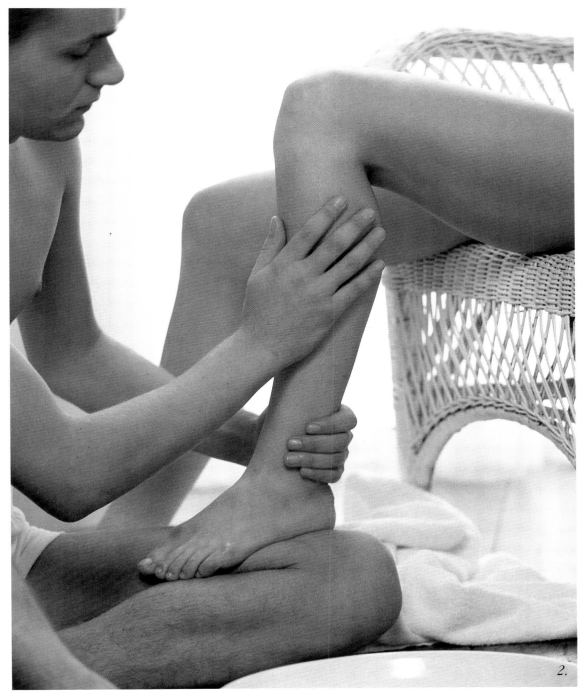

2.

2. Spread oil or lotion on the leg and start the massage with a series of smooth, flowing strokes on the lower leg to warm and relax the muscles responsible for moving the toes. With your fingers pointing to your partner's head, sweep your hands one after the other over the front of her leg to just below the knee. Glide your hands to the back of the leg and, moulding them into the calf, pull them gently down to the back of her ankle. Sweep your hands around the ankle and repeat the stroke in an unbroken motion four times to boost the lymph and blood circulation.

3. Now do three flowing sequences of fan stroking up the leg from the ankle to just below the knee in much the same way as the fan strokes are performed on the thigh area on page 37. Make sure that your hands fully encompass the shape of her leg, so that as they fan out and around, your fingers stroke down behind the calf muscles before returning to the front of her leg. Feel her calf muscles ripple and loosen beneath your strokes.

4. Support the ankle with your left hand and apply pressure to the fingers of your right hand to stretch into the tissue along the outer ridge of your partner's shin bone. As it reaches the knee, sweep it back down behind her leg while your left hand repeats the motion on the inner ridge of the shin bone. As each hand reaches the back of the heel, slide your fingers firmly around the ankle bone before your hand ascends the front of the leg. Repeat the sequence three times.

5. Knead the muscles on the back of her leg by placing your right hand over her calf, gently lifting and squeezing the flesh between your fingers and heel and then releasing the pressure. Knead down the leg from just below the back of her knee to the Achilles tendon of the heel.

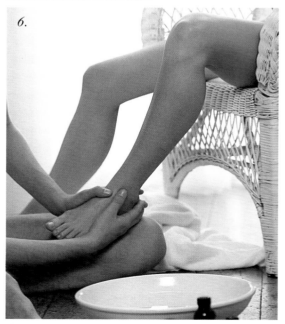

6. The ankles bear the pressure of the whole body weight and are put under strain when there are problems with posture. Stiff ankle joints inhibit

movement and can make the whole body feel unsupported from ground level. Soaking the ankles in warm water and then massaging them to ease tension held around the joints will increase suppleness in the feet and bring relaxation to the whole body structure, including an aching back. Use the fingertips of both hands to sweep deftly around and around the outer edges of the anklebones. Then lightly cup your hands behind her ankle so your fingers are interlaced. Use your thumb pads to massage thoroughly, one thumb following the other in small outward-moving circles over the front of the ankle. This movement is made by rotating the base thumb joint, and is more effective if pressure is applied on the upward and outer half of the circle with a softer glide back. Once you have massaged the sides and front of the ankle stroke all around each side of her heel with tiny fingertip circles, using both hands simultaneously.

7. Rub a little more lotion between your hands and slide both hands, fingers pointing towards the ankle, over the instep. Circle your fingers around her anklebones and draw your hands back down the sides of the foot to her toes so that your fingers stroke firmly along the sole of her foot. Repeat this movement four times without breaking the flow of motion and feel how her foot softens and warms beneath your touch.

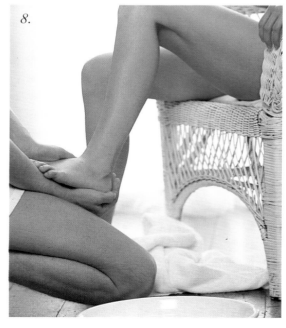

8. Rest her heel in your right hand and place the fingers of your left hand under the sole of her foot. Rotate the heel of your hand all over the outer half of the instep and alongside the heel while your fingers simultaneously massage the sole of her foot. Then pass the foot to your left hand and massage in the same way on the inner side of the instep and heel with your right hand.

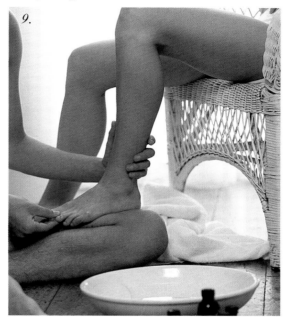

9.

9. Toes, which are usually cramped and tense, appreciate a gentle stretch, combined with movement and massage. Start with the little toe and clasp it above and below the base joint with your thumb and index finger. Gently rotate the first joint three times in both directions and then slide along to the top joint and wiggle it up and down. Go back to the base joint with your thumb and finger and pull firmly but sensitively along the toe. Give a firm squeeze to the tip of the toe before snapping your fingers out of it. Repeat these movements on the other toes. You will need to swap the position of your hands to stretch along the last two toes.

10. The skin on the sole of the foot is usually quite thick, so increase the pressure of your strokes as you massage its surface. Rest the heel of her foot in your left hand. Now clasp the foot with your right hand so that your fingers lie across the instep and your thumb is on the sole, just below the flat of the heel. Move your thumb in short, firm strokes, one slide

following another, to cover the area from the heel to the base of the toes. Then make a loose fist with your hand and grind your knuckles in small semi-circular actions all over the sole, keeping a check that the pressure is not too hard.

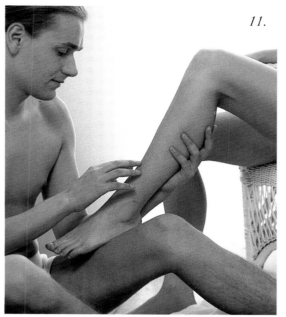

11.

11. Light feather stroking down the leg and foot with your fingertips, one hand overlapping the other, will give the massage a stimulating skin-teasing finish. To increase the skin sensation further, gently rake over the top of her foot with your fingernails. Then cradle the foot between your hands for several moments.

12. Dry the left foot, remove the bowl, and repeat all of the above strokes. When you have finished the massage, lift both feet to rest the soles softly on the surface of your belly. Breathe into your abdomen and imagine that you are sending your breath out into your partner's feet. She will enjoy feeling the rise and fall of your belly as you breathe beneath her feet.

THE EFFECTS OF FOOT MASSAGE

Foot massage can produce a calming and soporific effect on the physical system or an invigorating one. Soft strokes will reduce anxiety and induce a good sleep. A gentle foot massage is a perfect antidote to stress and insomina, while more vigorous strokes and deeper pressure will boost a sluggish system.

A w a k e n i n g
the senses
to love

Human beings have a tremendous capacity for experiencing pleasure

through the five senses of sight, sound, smell, taste and, above all, touch.

Heightening these senses to the point of exquisite joy is a playful art

which can bring a new and deeper level of intimacy between two

people in a loving relationship.

THIS CHAPTER encourages you to make time in your relationship to create a shrine to love, pleasure and the five senses of the body. It suggests ways to involve and heighten all the senses, so that one sensation merges and expands into another in a shared experience of mutual trust and exploration. By opening the doors of your sensory awareness to taste, smell, sight, sound and touch you will be able to honour your own body and that of your partner, and allow them to become what many Eastern mystics have long called the human body – 'the temple of the spirit'.

PREPARING THE ALTAR OF LOVE
Take time to prepare the ambience for your sensual experience so that it becomes a total celebration of the awakening of all five senses. Choose an after-noon or evening when both of you can relax into a long period of uninterrupted pleasure. Everything that you do in this time should resonate with the feeling of opulence, beauty, romance and sensation.

Heightening your sensory awareness will turn each tender touch into an act of worship.

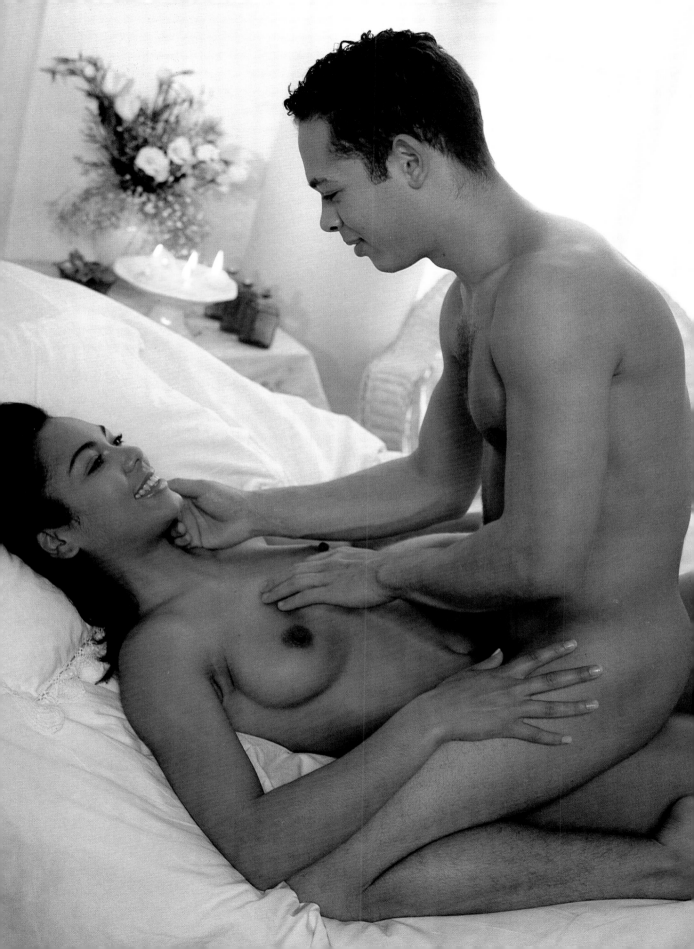

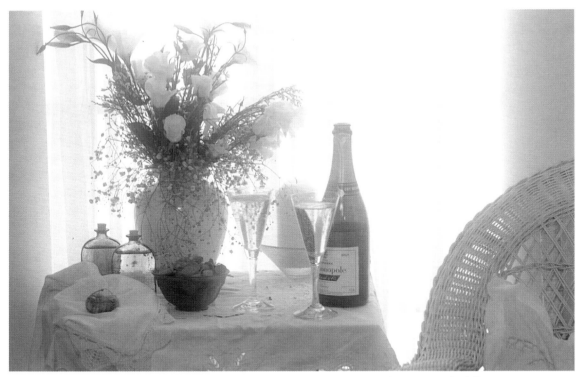

Prepare your room for the sensual massage before the event as if you are creating an altar for love. You are, after all, setting the scene for an act of worship of your partner's body. The very fact that you have taken time to consider all aspects of the giving of pleasure will be appreciated by your lover as an indication of your deep regard.

The first thing to do is to clear away any clutter from the room so that you have plenty of space to move freely, in addition to making the environment visually restful. Place vases of beautiful flowers such as roses, lilies and freesias around the room to delight the eye. Warm the room to a minimum of 75°F/24°C. Remember that your partner will be lying still and her body temperature may drop while yours heats up by virtue of your being active. Many of your sensual strokes will flow over the entire body, so it is preferable that your partner is naked and uncovered. However, keep some warm towels or a soft blanket nearby to cover her if she starts to feel cold. Always be prepared to take your partner's modesty into consideration and, if necessary, allow him or her to remain partially clothed. You may have to adapt your strokes, but if you respect your partner's wishes, trust will develop and it will not

To enjoy a sensual massage to the full, turn your room into a shrine of love, choosing items to bedeck it that will stimulate and enhance all five senses.

be long before any initial inhibitions are shed.

Pick a firm but comfortable surface to work on. The bed is the most obvious choice, but some mattress and bed bases are too soft to support the body fully under the pressure of certain strokes. You also need plenty of room to manoeuvre while you perform the massage so that you cause the least disturbance to your partner. You may want to put the mattress on the floor, or you can use a piece of foam, a sleeping bag or folded up blankets. Make sure that, if you are working at floor level, you have padded support, such as cushions and pillows, to sit and kneel on while you give the massage.

Remember that everything you prepare in the room should aim to please the visual, olfactory, aural and touching senses. Cover the massage base with warm, clean and soft-to-the-touch sheets of harmonious colour tones. The lighting should be low and seductive and must never shine directly into your partner's eyes. Light candles around the room for a romantic ambience and to throw complimentary shadows flickering over the skin. For sound, choose soft mellow music or favourite tunes that evoke fond memories. Select whatever pleases the ear but keep the volume low so that it does not invade your massage or feelings but lulls you both into a relaxed, sensual and euphoric mood.

To stimulate your taste buds along with your other senses during the massage, keep a bottle of champagne or wine or a jug of tropical fruit juices close by to drink in moments of rest and playful exchange. Sip it and slowly let the liquid roll around the tongue so that its flavour is fully savoured. To delight your sense of smell, fill the room with delicate aromatic perfumes that induce a mood of euphoria, relaxation, harmony, earthiness, sens- uality, sexiness and emotional openness. Do this by placing aromatic potpourri in bowls, burning good incense sticks or lighting special burners filled with seductively perfumed essential oils, so that the fragrance fills the whole room. If you choose pot- pourri, select sweet-smelling petals of bright, sexy and luscious colours such as reds, pinks, blues, mauves and lilacs that will appeal to the eye as well as the nose. Alternatively, make a recipe of suitable essential oils to blend with your basic carrier oil and use it to anoint your partner's skin as an integral part of the loving massage.

It is important to choose the smells carefully so that they do not conflict or become overpowering. To combine the right ingredients for a sensual and seductive blend of oils, select one of the five aromatic essential oil recipes listed in the next chapter. Study the properties of the oils and then choose the most appropriate blend for yourself and your lover. Each mixture will influence your mood so that your uninhibited sensuality and eroticism can emerge. They will also encourage relaxation, playfulness, calmness and joy. Pour the blended oils into a glass or porcelain dish or bottle and place it where it cannot be knocked over.

Depending on how you wish to use your essential oils, follow the recipes in the next chapter carefully so that you add just the right ingredients to your massage oil or aromatherapy burner, or even to a bath for a luxurious soak for two prior to the sensual feast of touch and massage.

SENSUAL MASSAGE

A sensual massage is an exercise in the pure pleasure of giving and receiving touch with no other goal in mind. Yet, naturally, when massage is experienced between lovers, the border between sensuality and sexuality merges, and the only rule is that the massage must be given in an atmosphere of mutual trust and agreement as to where touch purely for sensual pleasure ends and the shared enjoyment of eroticism begins.

In this chapter we explore sensual massage for its own sake, though all of the strokes combine to make the basis of an erotic massage as well. A sensual massage has its own profound benefits when it is given and received without any expectation of a consequent sexual act. It is very rare that we are able to simply open ourselves up to being pleasured and touched with reverence and love, to enjoy the interplay of sensual and sexual feelings within our own bodies, without some subtle demand of res- ponse and action. Learning to give and receive sensual massage can enhance a relationship in many ways. It helps lovers become deeply familiar with one another's bodies in a way that the sexual act alone cannot. No part of the body is left neglected as every inch is explored with a range of touch, from lingering caresses with the fingertips to tantalize the skin surface to deeper pressure from the hands to ease and soothe away muscular tensions. The back of the knees, under the arms, the tip of the nose, the legs, the arms, the body and face – all are equally revered with a loving touch.

Sensual massage is therefore a perfect tool to be used within a relationship whenever there are sexual anxieties because it enables a couple to explore and expand the parameters of their physical intimacy without immediate sexual pressure. Through caring and sensitive touch, a person can relax and awaken to sensual pleasure at his or her own pace. In discovering that the body is worthy of being loved and respected purely for its own sake, the inner emotional needs are met and nourished and trust begins to build. In times of stress or sexual dysfunction when, for whatever reason, sexual intercourse becomes difficult or impossible, then a loving sensual massage can remove frustration and create a physical bonding.

THE PLEASURE AND CREATIVITY IN GIVING MASSAGE

When you receive a sensual massage in a warm and carefully prepared setting where every sense of the body is heightened and cherished, the experience feels like a true gift of love. Yet to give a sensual massage is also an enlightening experience, because it enables you to access and share your inner resources. It helps you to grow in confidence about yourself as a sensuous and feeling person. In the process of learning how and where to touch your partner's body and in witnessing what pleasure this brings, you gain trust in your own intuitive responses to another's needs and in your ability to give comfort and joy.

A whole range of feelings can be transmitted through the physical contact of your hands on your partner's body, allowing the expression of many aspects of your personality regardless of your gender. You can stroke your partner with the tenderness of a parent to a child, cherish him or her with touches that only a lover can impart, massage and release away pain and tension with hands that are strong, protective and skilful, or discover the childlike wonder in yourself as you play with his or her body.

You can turn your massage into a creative art. Your hands may move like liquid over the shape and form of your loved one's body, flowing like water to encompass every curve and dimension. Through your strokes, your partner will come to realize the intrinsic beauty of his or her body. Your hands may touch the skin with the softness of silk, the lightness of a feather, the suppleness of a sculptor and the dexterity of a craftsperson.

Let your massage become a dance of the hands, changing at a rhythmic pace from one motion to another, gliding over the trunk or the limbs of the body in long sweeping and rounded strokes, fanning outwards or in circles. Slide your hands to integrate the various body parts with soothing stretches, bringing a sense of unity and connection from head to toes. Alternatively, your hands can rest with

During a sensual massage even the subtlest of touches, such as the light brush of hair against the skin, will enliven the skin senses.

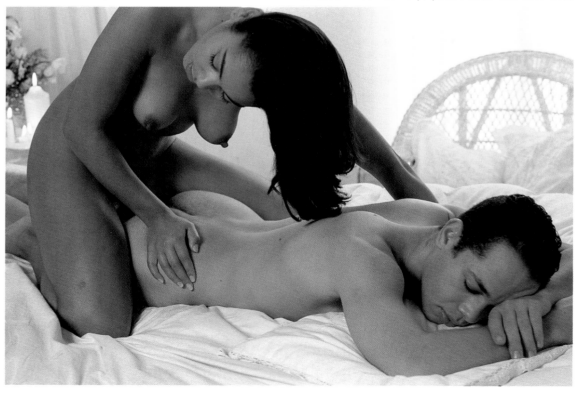

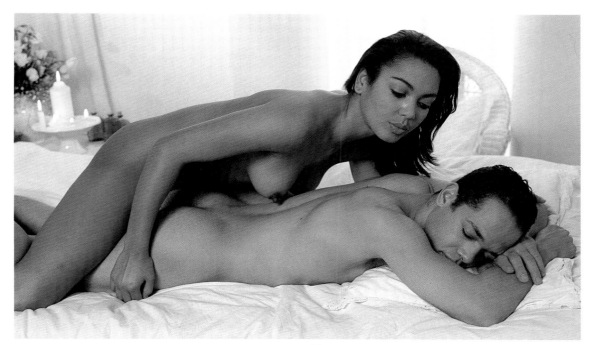

In an atmosphere of mutual trust and caring, every part of the body can become fully involved in the play of a sensual massage.

exquisite stillness over the head, the heart, the belly or the feet and by their very presence impart a calm and healing touch.

When you are massaging your partner, use not only your hands to make contact but any part of your body that is comfortably able to touch, caress and stroke. Bring as much of yourself into the massage as possible. Don't just stroke with your hands – stroke with your forearms too. If you have long hair, let it fall and sweep over the skin. This works wonderfully when you are returning the movement back down the body. First your partner will feel the comforting pressure of your hands as they move up the body, soothing and stretching away tension from the soft tissue, then the gentle slide, raking or feathering of your hands and fingers as they draw back down, followed by the barely felt and teasing brush of your hair. Use your breath to blow softly over areas that have just been massaged so that its warmth feels like a subtle breeze whispering over the skin. These different levels of pressure awaken the skin's vast network of sensory nerve receptors.

KEEPING THE MASSAGE SENSUAL

When the massage is focused purely on sensuality and is not aimed at progressing towards eroticism – or if you both wish to delay sexual excitement and linger for as long as possible on the tantalizing border where one merges into the other – there are a few things to remember. While a sensual massage can, and indeed should, encompass all body parts, including the genitals and breasts, if either of you is becoming aroused you should gently move away from these areas so that sexual excitement is diffused back into a soft stream of sensual feeling. Slide from the thighs over the genitals and on up to the belly and chest, or glide your hands down the legs to massage the feet. Cup and caress the breasts but then stroke on over the whole chest, or up around the shoulders and over the neck, head and face. Relax into giving and receiving touch entirely for its own sake, letting go of thoughts, fantasies and desires that race ahead towards a sexual goal. Take your time to give the massage if your partner is clearly enjoying it. A whole body massage can last for an hour or even longer – there is no hurry and nothing to do except to relish the sheer ecstasy of awakening the sense of touch, the abandonment to pure sensuality, and the playful devotion to your partner's body.

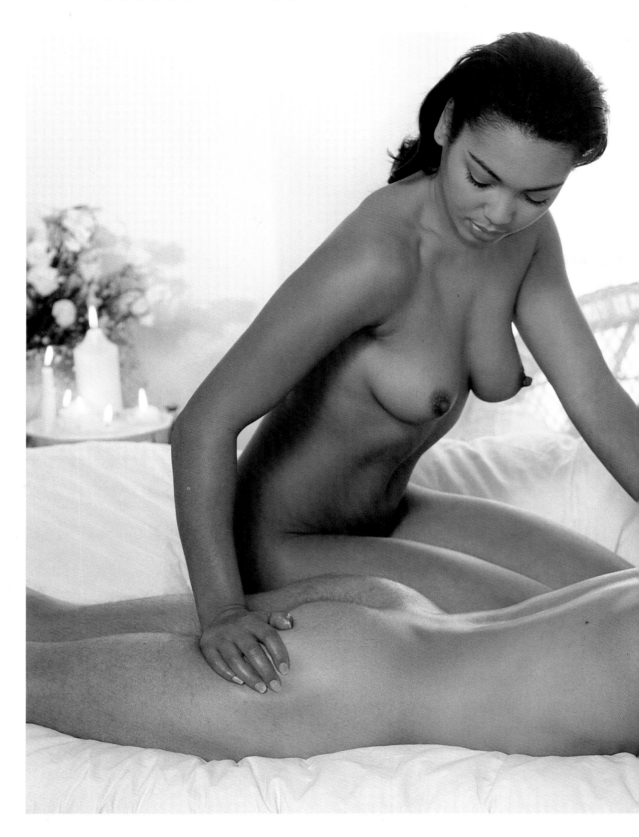

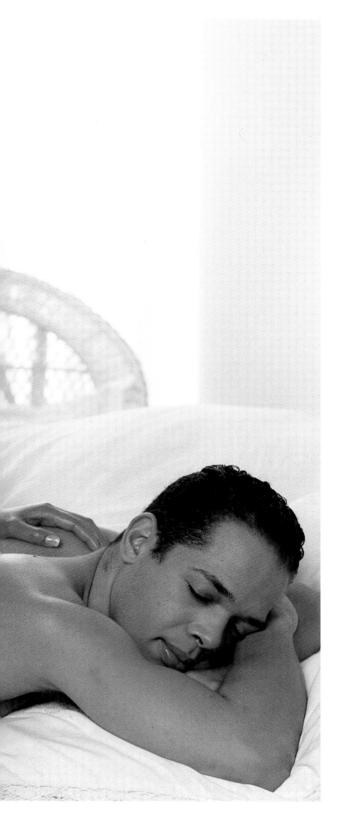

MASSAGING THE BACK OF THE BODY

1. Help your partner to undress and find a comfortable position lying face down on the mattress. Give him a little time to settle and relax, and while he is doing so place your hands softly over the top and base of his spine. Take some moments to become aware of your own breathing, letting go of your thoughts, expectations and goals so that you are able to be totally in the present moment, available to dedicate all of yourself to giving this massage with love and respect.

2. Rub a little oil into your hands and begin to spread it first over his back, and then down his legs. During a therapeutic session, it is normal to spread oil only on the area that is to be massaged immediately. However, in a sensual massage, your hands need to move constantly over the whole length and shape of the body.

Lean your body weight into the strokes, finding a pressure that is both gentle and reassuring. Use your hands and also the soft skin surface of your forearms to spread oil over the back and sides of your partner's body. Let your hands flow in a constant rhythmic motion to explore and mould your lover's curves and contours, allowing your fingers to drift delicately into the crevices and folds of the body as the hands sweep by. Bring into your hands a sense of wonder at the mysteries of your partner's body. Allow them to become increasingly supple as if they are melting into the depth of the skin, embracing not only the muscles, tissue, joints and bones but the very essence of the person you love.

Spreading the oil is an integral part of a sensual massage and it helps you to become intimately familiar with the body. Make it a dance, using strokes that fan, circle and stretch soft tissue, warm the muscles and integrate the limbs and torso. This will allow time for your partner's breath to deepen while his body relaxes and becomes more alive and available to receiving your touch.

3. Rake and then feather stroke down the whole body so that the skin begins to tingle.

While spreading the oil in a sensual massage, let your hands play in a variety of soft, flowing strokes over the whole of your partner's body.

1.

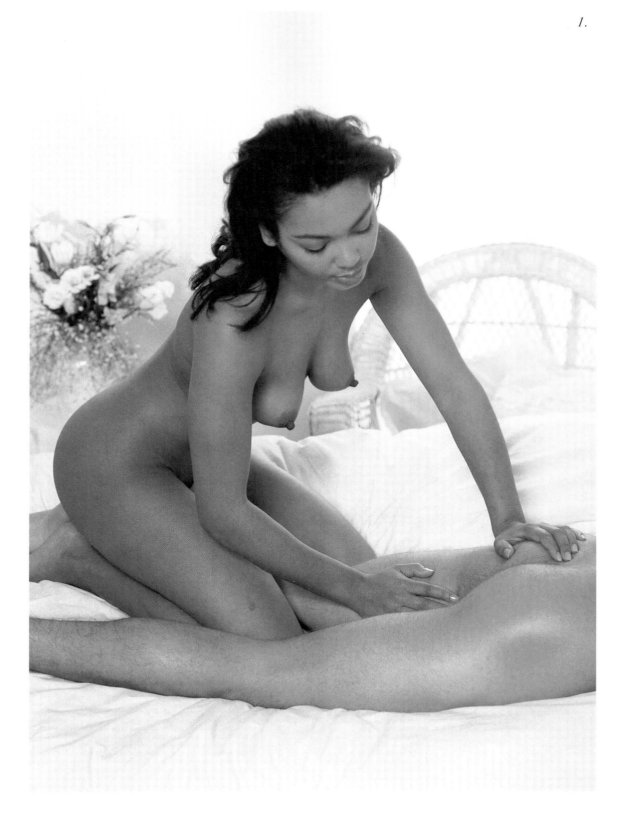

THE LEGS

1. You have covered the whole of the back of your partner's body with oil and loving touch and it is now time to focus on his legs. When massaging the legs, always include the buttocks, pelvis and hips in your strokes for a fully sensual and integrated effect. Kneel by your lover's foot and begin with a full flowing stroke that covers the entire area. Place both hands, fingers pointing towards the thigh, over the back of the ankle of the left leg. Slide with a firm, steady pressure upwards, softening your hands as they pass over the back of the knee. As your right hand reaches the top of the thigh, slip it sensitively onto the inner thigh just below the genitals. Let it wait there while the left hand continues up over the buttocks, fanning out around the pelvis and hip and returning down to the outer thigh. Without breaking the flow of motion, draw both hands firmly back down the leg to the ankle and repeat the sequence.

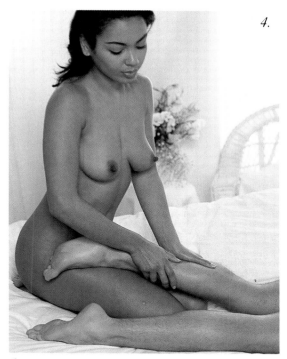

4.

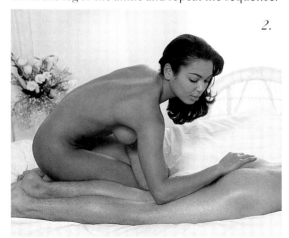

2.

2. Place your right hand across the ankle, little finger leading, and sweep it up the entire length of the left leg, fanning it over the buttocks and bringing it lightly down the right leg. Repeat this stroke several times, interchanging the surface of your hand and forearm to caress the skin.

3. Pick up your partner's left leg at the ankle to flex his knee so that his lower leg is slightly raised and resting across your knee. Stroke over his calf with both hands from the ankle to just below the back of the knee before fanning them out to the sides of his leg and gliding them back down and out over the foot. Repeat several times to relax and warm the calf muscles.

4. Now massage over the lower leg, with one hand following the other, in alternating fan strokes. The pressure is applied mainly from the heel and sides of the thumb, while simultaneously the fingers curl around and stroke over the front of the leg. When both your hands reach the back of your partner's knee, slide them down the sides of his leg. Circle your fingers around his ankle bone, then swivel your hands back to their original position. Repeat the sequence twice more.

5. To knead the lower leg, sit or kneel to face it and place both hands, several inches apart, over the calf so that your fingers are pointing towards the other leg. Knead thoroughly up and down over the muscles.

6. Change your position so that once again you can make the long sweeping strokes which cover first the calf and then the whole of the leg. Stop at some point to linger lovingly over the back of your partner's knee, as this area is surprisingly sensitive and receptive to touch. Let your hands sensuously fan stroke over its softness with the lightest of touches. Then trail your fingertips over its surface, decreasing the pressure until they are making subtle contact. Finally, lean forward to send the caress of your breath gently over the skin.

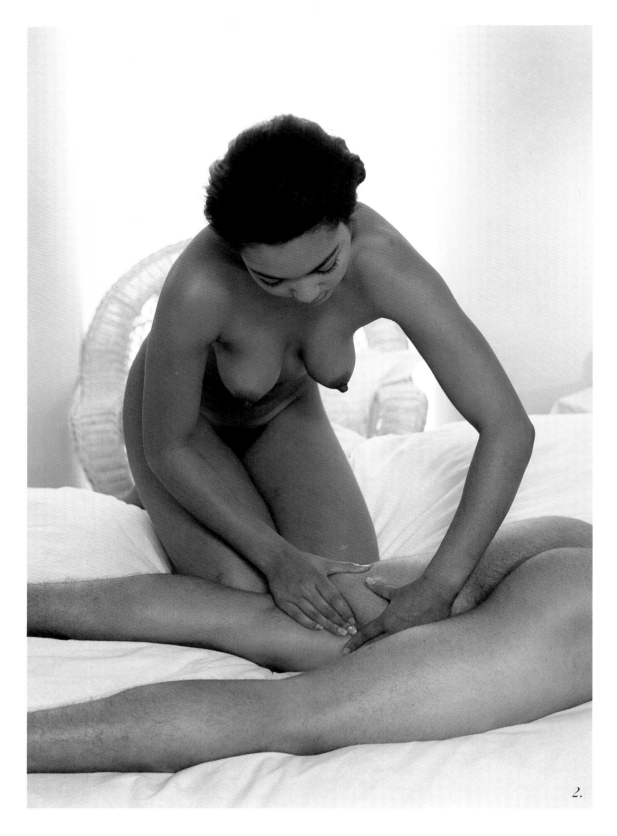

2.

UPPER LEG AND BUTTOCKS

1. Bring your attention to the thigh and buttocks, so that your massage soothes and stimulates the muscles which surround the genitals. Let your tender stroking play on the fine border between sensual and sexual arousal as your hands slip onto the inner thigh, under the fold where the buttocks meets the leg, and gently along the groin. Cover the thigh and buttocks with strokes that embrace its full shape. Use fan strokes, circle strokes and alternate fanning.

2. Knead thoroughly over the inner thigh, then the front and outer side of the thigh and up onto the the buttocks, lifting and rolling the flesh between your hands.

3. When you have finished kneading, slide your hands apart over your partner's thigh in a long, soft stretch so that your left hand swims up over the length of his back while your right hand moves down the leg and stops on the foot. Let your left hand encircle the shoulder and continue down the

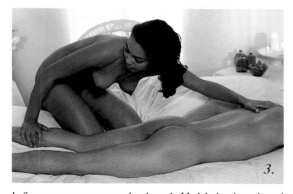

3.

left arm to rest over the hand. Hold the hand and foot for some moments with stillness and calm so that your lover can feel the connection between the different parts of his body under your caring touch.

4. Rake and then feather touch from the lower back, over the buttocks and down both legs and feet. Sweep your hair over the lower body and then blow your breath softly over the skin, focusing it like a warm breeze over the buttocks. Repeat all of the leg and buttocks strokes on the right side of the body.

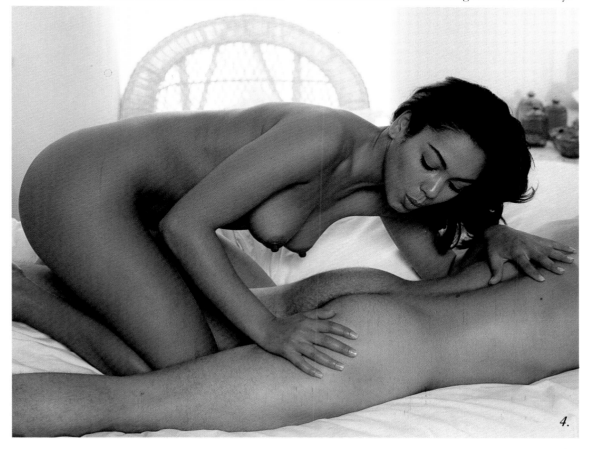

4.

THE BACK

1. Straddle your partner's thighs, keeping one foot on the mattress so that you are able to lever yourself back and forth as you massage the length of his back. Your inner thighs can press gently against your lover's skin, but support your own weight rather than allowing it to drop down onto his body. Now spread a little more oil on his back with sweeping, rounded strokes, again emphasizing the shape of the body.

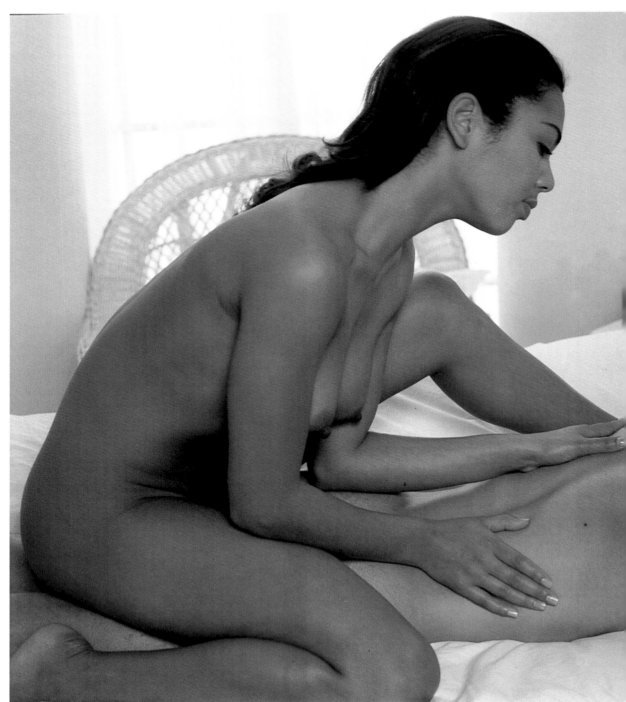

2. Place your hands flat on the lower back, fingers pointing towards the head, to rest on each side of the spine. Glide both hands with a soft, firm pressure along the length of the spine, easing away tightness from the muscles that support the vertebrae. Fan

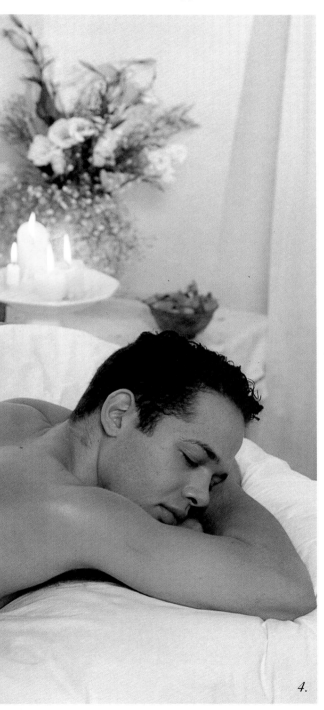

4.

your hands out over his shoulders and down along the sides of the ribcage. When your hands reach his waist, slide them lightly around and back towards the spine so that you can repeat this main back stroke twice more.

3. Fan stroke up the back, remembering to mould your hands into the sides of the ribcage as they draw back down. As you reach the upper back, expand the fanning shape to embrace the shoulders before pulling your hands down the sides of his body and back to the base of the spine. Repeat twice more.

4. Increase the pressure in your hands to ease away tension from the lower back with a series of alternate fan strokes. With one hand following the other, work up each side of the spine to just below the shoulder blades before drawing back down the sides of the body.

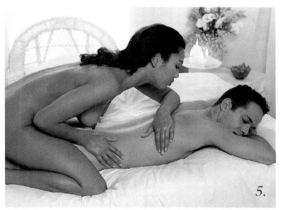

5.

5. Lean towards the body so there is close physical contact and cover the back with broad, sweeping circles, using the surface of your forearms. Then place both forearms parallel across the lower back. Drop your weight gently into the pressure as you push your forearms steadily up over the back. When you reach the upper back, spread your hands out over the shoulders and arms.

6. If your weight is not too heavy, softly cover your partner's body with your own, so that your chest and belly form a protective blanket of love over his skin. Relax and breathe together, allowing your bodies to melt into one another. Feel yourself expanding with the inhalation of breath and sinking together with the exhalation as the breathing synchronizes; experience its rise and fall as a wave washing over you.

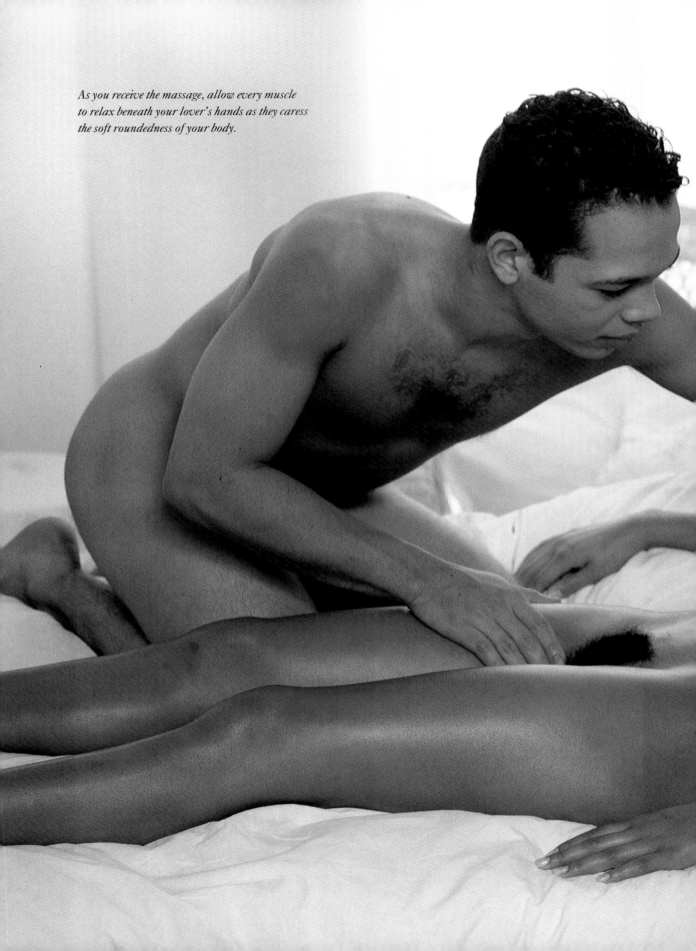

*As you receive the massage, allow every muscle
to relax beneath your lover's hands as they caress
the soft roundedness of your body.*

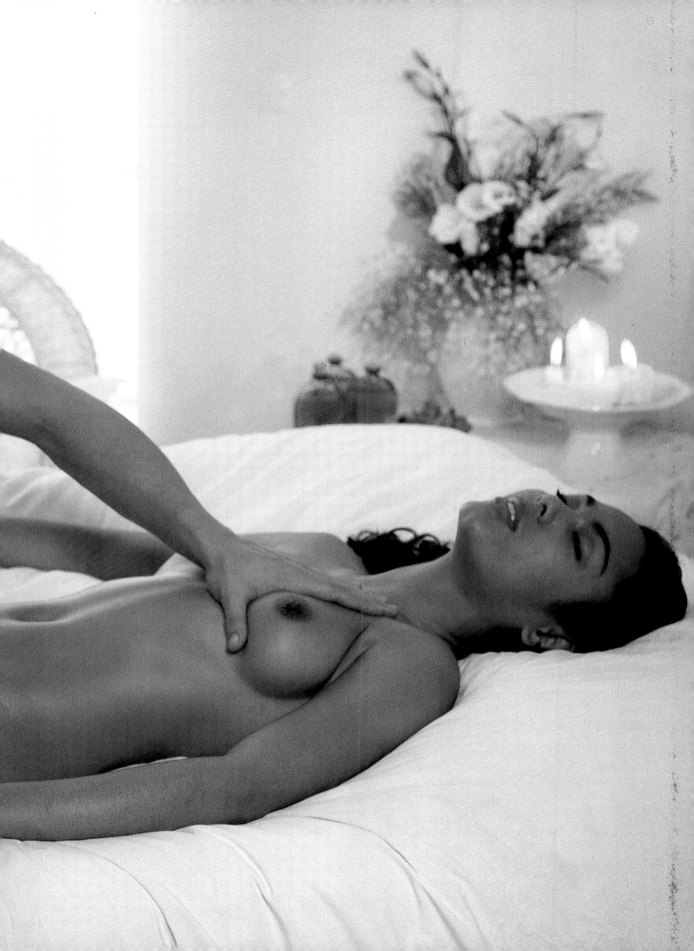

THE FRONT OF THE BODY

The front of the body is obviously quite different anatomically and psychologically to massage than the back. As your partner turns over, even greater sensitivity is needed in the intention of your touch. As tension eases and the senses expand, soft and vulnerable feelings emerge which need to be cherished with every loving touch. Many of the strokes and sequences over the front of the body are similar to those you have already performed on the back, but your hands will need to acknowledge the different curves and contours, the shape and sensitivity of the breasts, the softness of the belly, the delicacy of the face and the intimacy of the genitals.

1. Kneeling by your partner's abdomen, place your left hand over her heart and your right hand over her lower belly. Merge with your partner through touch and breath. Then spread oil over the chest, belly, legs and arms. Let your hands fan out in free-flowing movements over the surface of the skin to embrace their rounded dimensions. As you stroke over the front, integrate its various parts in long unbroken motions, hands spreading apart and circulating with great fluidity from one area to another.

Pour all of yourself into your touch so that your hands become finely tuned, picking up the body messages and acknowledging the underlying feelings. Fan and circle stroke as appropriate, sliding into long stretches. Lean over the body for close physical contact, using the broad surface of your forearms to sweep the skin. Include the intimate areas of the breasts and genitals in your strokes as your hands sweep sensitively by, but do not linger on these zones. Complete your strokes by taking them around and out of the body.

THE FEET, LEGS AND BELLY

Start to focus your sensual strokes on specific areas of the body, starting with the feet and legs and then moving onto the abdomen. Combine the free-flowing movements and teasing touches with other strokes given in the previous chapters of this book. For the feet, use strokes from the Foot Massage (page 58), flowing on up the legs with movements described in Relaxing the Thighs and Groin

(page 37). Infuse your hands with love as you change position to face the abdomen and continue with the Belly Massage programme (page 36). Kneading strokes can be integrated into your massage over the fleshy areas such as the thighs, hips and sides of the waist.

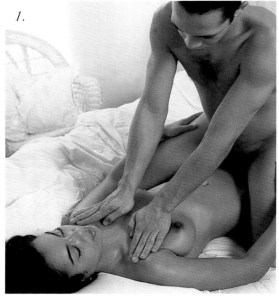

1.

THE CHEST AND ARMS

1. Kneel by your partner's waist so that you face towards her head. Rub a little oil into your hands, and slide them, fingers close together and pointing towards the neck, up over the breastbone. Fan them out under the collarbone towards each shoulder, leaning your weight into the stroke to release tension from the muscles and increase the breath. This will allow the chest to expand so that the vulnerable feelings that are held in that area can emerge. Let your hands slip around her shoulders and onto the sides of her ribcage just below the armpits. Wrap your hands over the sides of her body so that your fingers stroke under her back as you pull them down to the base of her ribs. Swivel your wrists to stroke your hands back across to her breastbone and repeat the sequence again.

The combination of your tender touch, the release of her tension and the increase in her breath may bring your lover's emotions flowing to the surface. Be sensitive and caring if tears of sadness or joy begin to come, and allow her to experience her feelings.

2.

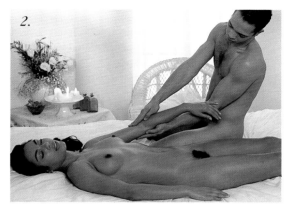

2. Kneel by your partner's left hand and spread the oil from the centre of her chest, over her shoulder and down both sides of her arm in gentle, over-lapping movements. Now sandwich the top of her arm between your hands, and pull slowly down its whole length to pass out of the hands and fingers.

3.

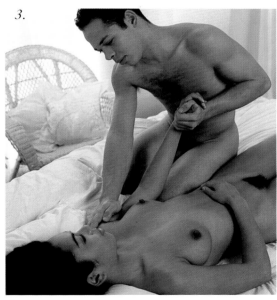

3. Soothe her arm with long, flowing and sensuous strokes that enliven the skin and revitalize the circulation. Hold her left hand with your right one and lay your left hand across her wrist, little finger leading. Stroke up over the front of her arm with your left hand, encircling her shoulder and gliding down the back of her arm to the wrist. Swap hands, and stroke along the inner arm to just below the armpit before circling round to return to the wrist. Continue to stroke over her arm, passing it from one hand to the other, until it feels completely relaxed.

4.

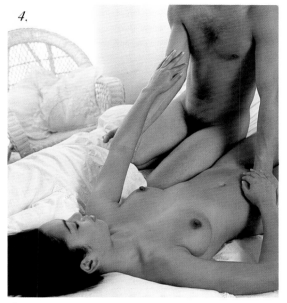

4. For maximum skin contact between you and your partner, place her left hand on your right shoulder, resting her arm along the soft inner surface of your own right arm. Slowly draw your hand down along her arm so that it falls softly towards the mattress. Trail your hand gently out over her palm so that your touch lingers on her fingertips.

5. Invigorate the arm with some of the strokes that you have used on other parts of the body, adapting the movement to suit its narrower structure. Massage from her wrist to her shoulder with three sequences of alternating fan strokes, passing her arm from one hand to the other to support the motion. Then raise her forearm, rest it on the elbow and hold the wrist in your right hand. Wrap your left hand just above the wrist and drain towards her elbow with a firm pressure. Lift her elbow to circle your fingers behind it before stroking back down her arm. Knead and stroke her upper arm, always completing your strokes by circulating your hands around her shoulder and back down to her elbow before repeating them. Complete these strokes with full-length motions, sliding up and back down the whole arm.

6. Rake your fingers in overlapping strokes down the arm from the shoulder to the hand. Follow this movement with teasing feather-light touches by brushing your fingertips right down the length of the arm.

THE HAND

1. From this position it is easy to massage her hand, adapting the strokes from the Hand Massage programme described on page 23. You can also work thoroughly over the palm by gently flexing her hand back at the wrist. Support the back of her hand with your fingers, using your thumb pads to stroke over the palm in tiny alternate circles, one thumb following the other.

2. To complete the chest, arm and hand massage, raise her arm slightly so that the elbow is flexed and resting on your knee. Lift her hand and place its palm over your heart. Let your right hand drop softly onto her chest so that it rests with great tenderness on her heart. Close your eyes and allow yourselves to merge into this heart-to-heart contact. Again, let the flow of your breath synchronize. Imagine it flowing between you through the contact of your hands.

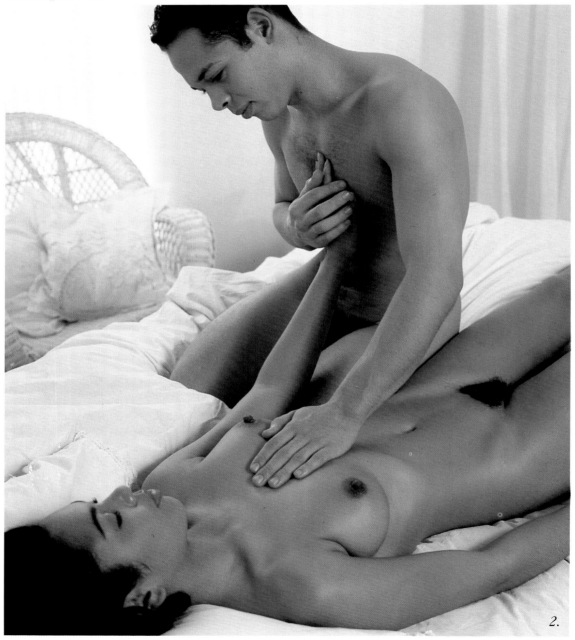

2.

THE FACE

Show your lover how much you treasure her by bringing the feelings of gratitude and appreciation into your hands as you caress the features of her face. Be totally present with every contact because nothing feels more personal, intimate and cherishing than to receive a loving and tender face massage. This sequence is made up of very soft and flowing strokes. Combine them with the healing and calming holds which are explained in A Face and Head Session on page 27. Very little lubrication is needed in a face massage, but a tiny amount of oil or lotion on your hands will ensure that your strokes are smooth and the skin is nourished.

1. Sit or kneel behind your partner's head, letting it rest between your thighs. You may want to place a thin pillow under her head to relax her neck. Ensure that your own posture is supported comfortably by pillows or cushions. Apply a small amount of oil or lotion to your hands and stroke with the lightness of silk up from her chest and over her neck and throat. Caress the jaw, one hand stroking after the other, on each side of her face, from the chin to the ear.

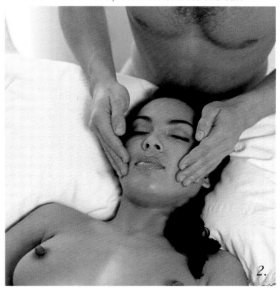

2. Cup both hands over her jawline so that your fingers meet on her chin. Stroke both hands up each side of her face to the top of the jaw before circling them around over the cheeks to softly slide back towards the chin. Continue this flowing motion until the jaw, cheeks and mouth relax beneath your hands.

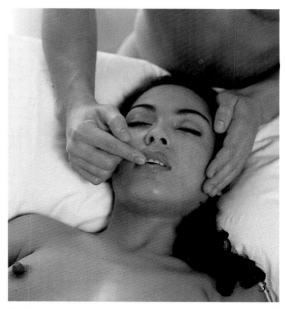

3. Using the tips of your fingers, gently massage all over both cheeks in tiny circles. Now, with the barest of touches, trace over the full softness of her lips with your fingertips.

4. The ears are very sensually responsive. Support the back of the ears with your fingertips and massage all over the lobes and edges with tiny thumb circles.

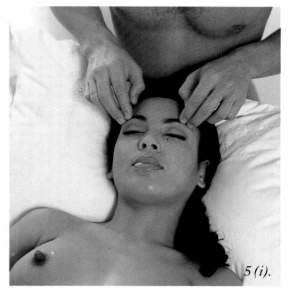

5 (i). Use the first two fingers of both hands to delicately circle several times around the eye-sockets. Placing them on the inner edges of the eyebrows, draw them out to the sides of the temples.

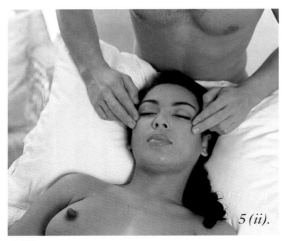

5 (ii).

5 (ii). Stroke your fingers back in over the cheek-bones towards the bridge of the nose. Lighten your touch as you stroke in towards her nose to avoid dragging the skin.

6. When you have made the last circle around her eyes, slide your fingers from the bridge of her nose down along its sides and then out over her cheek-bones to the sides of her face. Stroke around the temples several times.

7. Using the tip of a finger, brush very delicately over the ends of her eyelashes to create the subtlest of sensations.

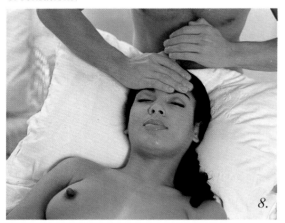

8.

8. Soothe her brow by placing your right hand across her forehead so that your fingers point towards the left. Brush your hand caringly up over the brow towards the hairline. Lift your hand slowly away from her head as you let your left hand softly drop down to repeat the motion. Stroke one hand after the other several times. Now run your fingers over her scalp, stroking out through her hair.

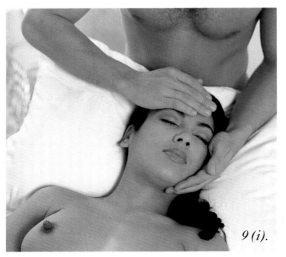

9 (i).

9 (i). Tilt her head so that it nestles into the support of your left hand. Place your right hand on her forehead so that your fingers point towards the left side of her brow.

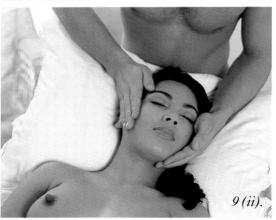

9 (ii).

9 (ii). Slide your hand over her brow and down onto the right side of her face, swivelling your wrist so that your fingers stroke down towards her chin.

9 (iii). Sculpt your hand so that it fits into the shape of her neck, fingers softly pointing towards the left side of the body, and gently stretch the muscles with the heel of your hand as you glide downwards to the shoulder.

9 (iv). Sweep around the shoulder, and stroke your fingers tenderly up over the back of the neck and through the hair. Do this sequence twice more before turning the head to the right and repeating the strokes. Complete by bringing her head back in line with the spine, and finish with a wonderfully calming series of face holds.

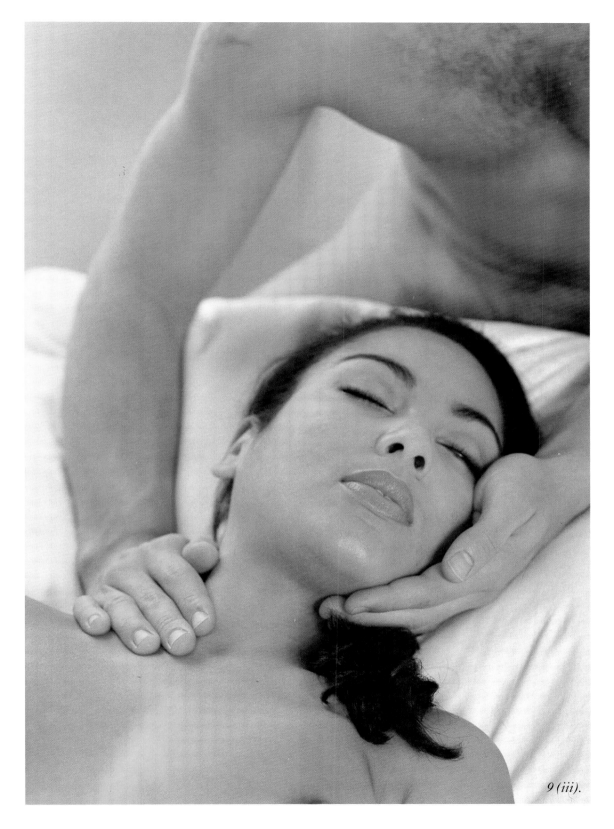

9 (iii).

COMPLETING A SENSUAL MASSAGE

What happens next now that you have adored the whole of your partner's body with lingering, loving and sensual touches will depend on the mutual feelings between you at that moment. You may want to cover your lover with a blanket and curl up beside her, enjoying the experience of being relaxed yet sensuously vibrant. If you received the massage, you can tell your partner how much you enjoyed being touched and how every moment of contact was precious to you. Let these moments be full of intimacy and appreciation for one another.

If the mood between you both during the massage became erotic, you may have included the more erogenous strokes and sequences that are shown in the next chapter. Your sensual massage may then have become a long and luxurious foreplay to making love.

SAFE SEX

Safe sex is essential to the art of love at the present time, as the HIV virus continues to spread throughout both homosexual and heterosexual populations. The virus can remain asymptomatic in an otherwise healthy person for many years, and any sexual act that involves contact with blood, semen or vaginal fluids puts lovers at risk of contracting it. Safe sex means taking adequate precautions against the exchange of these body fluids, and abstaining from high-risk sexual practices that involve such an exchange. The sensual and erotic massage programmes are safe sex practice. If you are making love with your partner in any way that involves penetrative sex, you should consider using condoms. If used correctly, condoms reduce the risk of catching the HIV virus and other sexually transmitted diseases. You may initially feel that condoms inhibit the spontaneity of love-making, but safe sex, like massage, is a way of showing how much you care for the well-being of the body, mind and spirit of both yourself and your lover.

When you have touched and cosseted every inch of your partner's body, relax together to savour fully these precious moments of rest and intimacy. Wait for another occasion to receive a sensual massage.

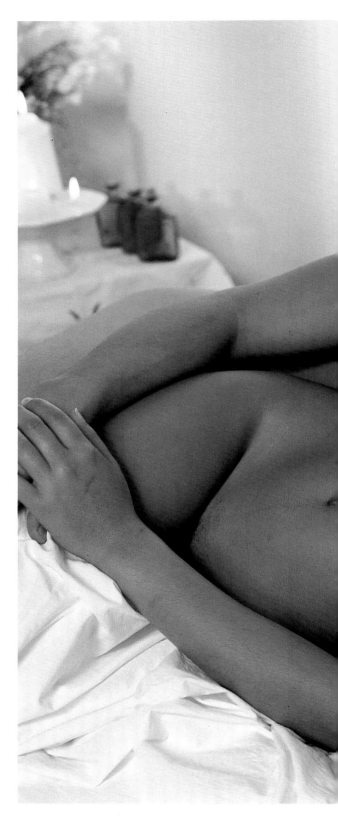

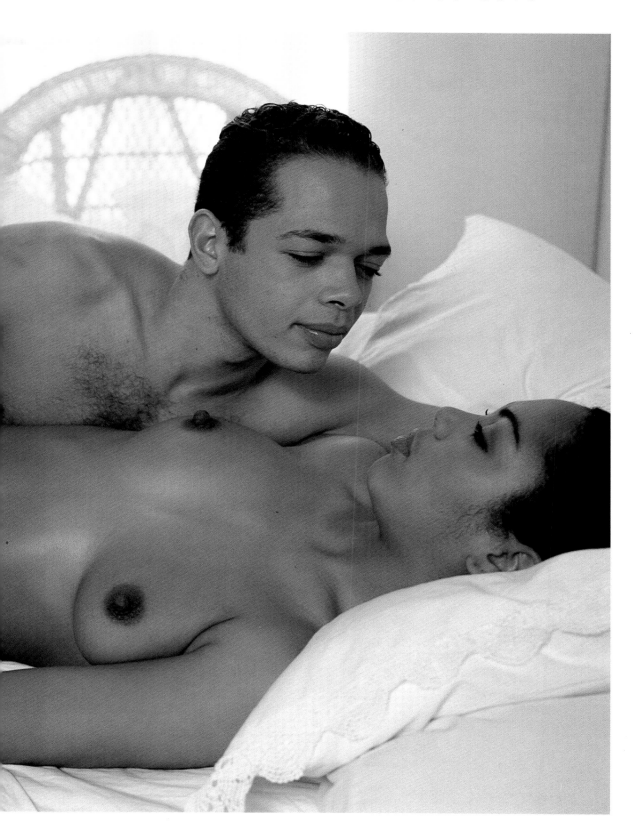

The erotic power of touch

Eroticism has been celebrated throughout history by many cultures. Paintings, poems, sexual practices and spiritual teachings have depicted eroticism as a creative act through which men and women can achieve sexual ecstasy and union.

THE ANCIENT TEMPLES of Khajuraho in India still draw thousands of people to admire their amazingly erotic wall sculptures. Likewise, the Kama Sutra has survived through the ages as a scripture on the joys of love-making. From the perfumed gardens and poetry of Persia to the teachings of Taoist Masters in China, the secrets of sexual pleasuring have been regarded by the ancients as a transcendental and mystical tradition.

Two thousand years ago in China, scholars taught the secrets of sexual happiness which they regarded as essential to achieving a healthy and balanced mind and body – yet earlier in this century, when the psychologist Wilhelm Reich (see Discovering The Orgasm Reflex, page 40) spoke of the link between sexual repression and neurosis he was condemned. Now, in the light of a more open attitude to sexuality, many people are seeking to rediscover the means to create deep emotional and physical satisfaction within a sexual relationship. Part of that process of exploration lies in unravelling the mysteries of the human body and its sexual geography.

Touch and massage, therefore, are the perfect tools for sexual foreplay. It is through the stimulation and stroking of the skin that sexually sensitive nerve receptors throughout the body are

Discovering the sexual geography of the body helps to deepen the physical and emotional bonding within a relationship.

86

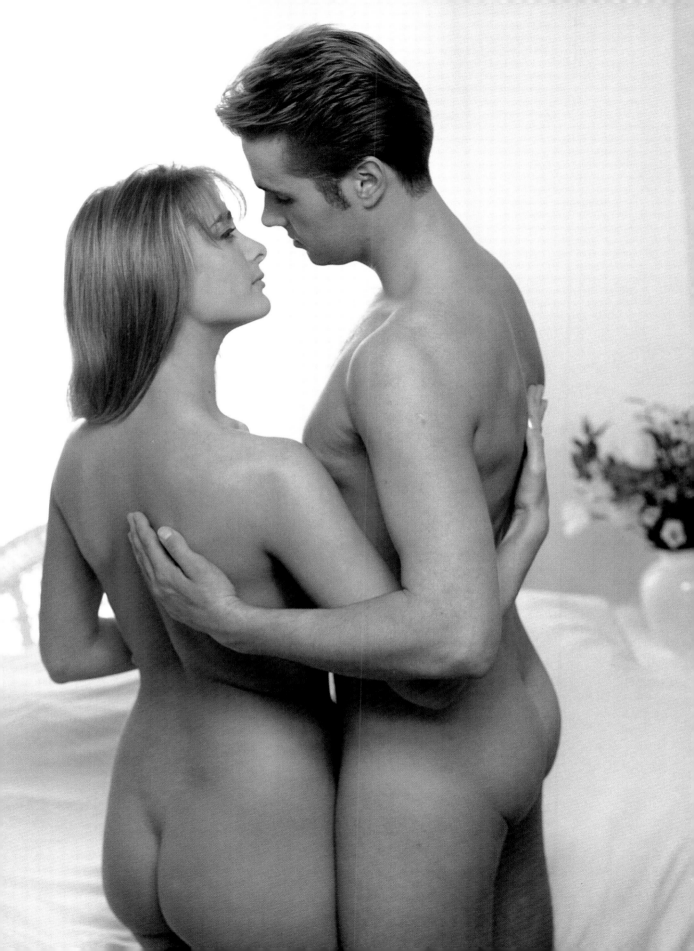

set alight. Sigmund Freud described the human body as being wholly erotogenic, and it is, indeed, through the skin that the tactile messages of love, tenderness and desire are received. By touching, caressing and fondling the skin, the flame of sexual desire is kindled, while at the same time the emotions and the soul are nourished.

PREPARING FOR AN EROTIC EXPERIENCE

SEXY FOOD

Eroticism can be manifested in many aspects of our lives. The way we move and dress, the colours we favour and how we decorate our homes can all enhance our experience of sensuality and eroticism – so pay attention to all the details as you prepare yourselves for a night of erotic massage.

Arousing your lover can begin at the dining table. Food and sex are fundamental to survival and the relationship between the two has been well documented. Prepare the meal to make it visually appealing, aromatically arousing and sensually pleasing to the tastebuds. Set the table with the most elegant cutlery and china that you possess, a lighted candle, and a vase of orchids, roses or deli-

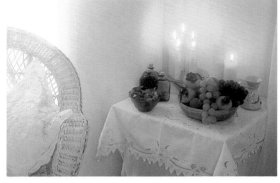

Fruit, flowers, aromatic oils and candles can all enhance eroticism when the mood is right. You can feed your lover delicious morsels of succulent fruit traditionally associated with sexuality.

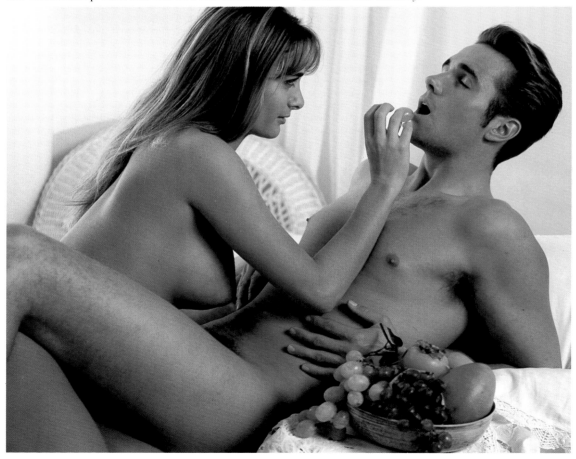

cate cut flowers. Choose food that is delicious and juicy but leaves you feeling light and energized. Pay special attention to selecting complementary combinations of colour, picking foods of rich rather than insipid hues. Certain foods – such as oysters, truffles, and chocolate – are said to have romantic and aphrodisiac qualities, while some spices have established sexual connotations. In India, garlic and onion are forbidden in some strict monastic communities because they are said to increase the libido!

Many fruits have been traditionally associated with sexuality, in some cases because their shape, colour and texture are suggestive of the male or female genital organs. In Greek myths, certain fruits were representative of the seed of life, symbolizing virility and fertility. Fruits such as pomegranates, figs and grapes were used in sacred temple rituals to signify the power of creation and regeneration, borne out in the sexual union of man and woman.

Prepare a cocktail of exotic fruits for your lover, choosing them for their sensual appeal – the mango, for instance, with its deep red colour, flowing juices and sensual fleshy texture, irresistibly evokes erotic images. Peel and cut the fruits into small pieces. Wait until his appetite is keen so his sense of smell and taste have increased. Ask him to close his eyes so he cannot see what you are popping into his mouth, and to focus his attention purely on the fragrance and taste of the fruits. Let him smell the fruits first before feeding him the delicious morsels piece by piece. He should take time to absorb their individual tastes, letting their sweetness melt in his mouth. He can lick their flavours from your fingers just as you can kiss away the juices from his lips.

AROMATHERAPY RECIPES FOR EROTICISM AND ROMANCE

Smell plays an important part in the enhancement of eroticism. Humans, like animals, are said to give off powerful sexual scents called pheromones from their sweat glands when they are in the mood for sexual activity. These odorous chemicals work subliminally and are believed to affect the behaviour of others without their even being aware of them.

For centuries, perfumers and apothecaries have used the essential oils of herbs, flowers and plants to create a similar sensual and erotic effect. These oils can be blended into potent recipes and, depending on the ingredients, produce a variety of remedial and sensual results. Smell affects not only the physical senses but the emotions too.

Here are five recipes to choose from if you wish to prepare an aromatic blend of oils for your erotic massage. Check the properties of the ingredients and follow the recipes carefully in order to create the mood best suited to you both:

	Massage *15 drops per 25 ml. base oil*	Aromatherapy Burner *7 drops*	Bath *7 drops*
1. Rosewood	7	3	3
Neroli	4	2	2
Rose	4	2	2
2. Ylang Ylang	8	3	4
Black Pepper	4	3	2
Patchouli	3	1	1
3. Rosewood	6	3	3
Lime	4	2	2
Jasmine	5	2	2
4. Frankincense	6	3	3
Bergamot	4	2	2
Sandalwood	5	2	2
5. Ylang Ylang	5	2	2
Patchouli	4	2	2
Mandarin	6	3	3

PROPERTIES FOR THE ESSENTIAL OILS

ROSEWOOD: Seductive, floral, woody fragrance. It steadies the nerves while being uplifting and calming. The sexy smell and calming combination help to ease sexual anxiety.

NEROLI: Haunting, bitter-sweet fragrance. It evokes feelings of peace, eases anxiety and is extremely sensual.

ROSE: Deep and luxurious, its floral perfume emits an exquisite and sensual aroma. It is often used to treat female reproductive disorders. Rose is said to help alleviate symptoms of sexual dysfunction such as impotence and frigidity. It has a calming effect and opens the heart up to tender feelings.

YLANG YLANG: This sweet, heady floral fragrance can aid relaxation and dissolve feelings of anger. It is said to alleviate sexual tension.

BLACK PEPPER: With its sweet peppery aroma, it adds a touch of spice and vitality. It is excellent for keeping your lover energetic and awake.

PATCHOULI: Its musky, exotic and earthy aroma adds a very sensual element to the recipe. It also calms the emotions, eases worry, and creates a meditative state of mind.

LIME: This has a sweet, mouth-watering smell and adds a light and playful energy to the blend.

JASMINE: A heady, exotic and deep lingering floral aroma which warms the emotions, gives extra confidence and dissolves lethargy. It is a very sensual and sexy oil for people who feel inexperienced, anxious, cold or tense.

FRANKINCENSE: A haunting, resinous, spicy perfume to create a meditative, calm and quiet mind, able to enjoy the moment rather than dwelling in the past.

BERGAMOT: A gorgeous, sweet and delicate odour which is very uplifting and relaxing. It helps to ease stress and adds a sense of joy to a lovers' blend.

SANDALWOOD: This is a sweet, woody and somewhat masculine fragrance which relaxes and eases stress and tension. It has long been reputed to have aphrodisiacal qualities.

MANDARIN: A fruity, tangy, citrus aroma which imparts a feeling of youthfulness and vitality that can add stamina to a night of love-making.

ADDING EROTICISM TO YOUR MASSAGE

By now you will know how to touch your lover in a therapeutic and sensuous manner – so it is time to use more than your hands to increase the eroticism of your massage! Intimate contact with your lover can be made not only by bringing your whole body into play, but by adding teasing and exciting stimulation with your lips, tongue and teeth. Each person's erotogenic response is unique and as you become familiar with your partner's body, you will find its secret pleasure places. Below are some suggestions focused on areas which usually have a high erogenous response. Naturally, as you stroke, rub, kiss, nibble, lick and gently suck on the sensitive skin, you will increase your own sexual

arousal as well. Do not over-focus on one particular area but constantly diffuse the sexuality so that it streams through the whole body. By combining this intimate contact with soft, tender strokes that spread all over the skin, the sexual sensations will constantly rise and fall, washing your lover in waves of ecstasy. The whole body will vibrate on a cellular level as you move from relaxation to excitation and back again. Try to avoid the temptation to rush headlong into heady excitement and penetrative sex – linger as long as you can in the exquisite joy of making love to your partner's body through massage and erotic touch.

While this chapter focuses on specific sexually sensitive zones, it is essential that you integrate those areas into a full body massage. Begin by using strokes to release tension and enliven the body, combining them with the flowing sensual massage motions given in the previous chapter. The full body integration stroke shown here is another wonderful way to embrace the whole body.

FULL BODY INTEGRATION STROKE

OVER THE BACK

Kneel beside your partner's feet, one foot on the mattress with the knee flexed in order to give you stability and leverage with this long movement which flows up and then back down the entire length of the body. At some point, you may need to change your position to reach the top of the shoulders or to sweep back down to the feet again.

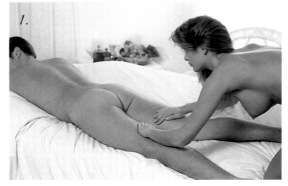

1. Place your hands across the back of each ankle, so that your fingers face inwards. Stroke both hands simultaneously up the legs, over the buttocks and onto the back, allowing them to mould into the body shape.

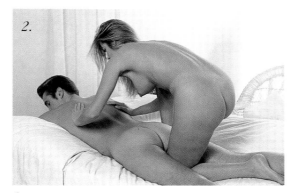

2.

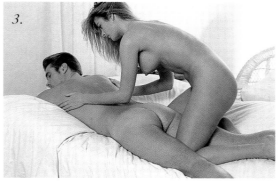

3.

2. Change your position if necessary. Support your own weight but lean forward so that your whole body makes close contact with your lover as your hands continue gliding up towards the shoulders. If possible, let your hair and breasts seductively brush against his skin to excite his senses.

3. Fan your hands out over his shoulders, and then slowly lever your own weight back onto your

haunches as your hands pull down the sides of his body.

4. Change position again, and let your fingers trail feather-light down his legs. Repeat this whole back of the body sequence three times so that your partner feels the surges of warmth, closeness and pressure with the upward flowing movement, and the gentle subsidence of the downward strokes.

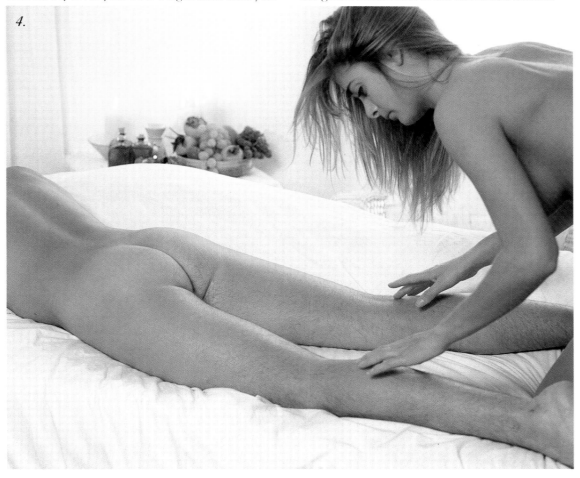

4.

1.

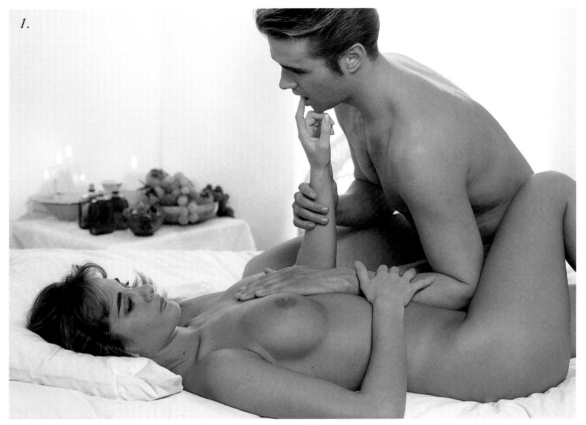

OVER THE FRONT

In a similar sequence of motions as on the back, you can integrate the front of the body to ensure a wonderful sense of unity. Be sure to soften your hands as they pass over the more delicate areas of the belly and chest.

Wrap your hands across the insteps of the feet, little fingers leading the stroke, to sweep up the front of the legs. Ease the pressure as you pass over the knees. Form your hands to the body as they pass over the hips and sides of the waist. Swivel your hands inwards, with fingers pointing towards the head to glide together up the breastbone and fan out over the pectoral muscles towards and around the shoulders. Softly stroke down the arms and hands, slipping back onto the legs to continue down to the feet. Turn your hands to wrap across the feet and repeat this lovely integration stroke. You can vary this stroke by returning your hands down along the sides of the body. By the end of these integration strokes, your partner will be wholly aware of her body from head to toes.

THE HANDS AND FINGERS

The fingertips, filled with thousands of sensory nerve endings, can be surprisingly responsive to erotic stimulation.

1. After relaxing your partner's arm with your sensual strokes and adapting the hand massage in Taking Hold of the Hands (page 22), her hand will feel alive and stimulated. Arouse your partner by placing each finger, one by one, into your mouth and massaging it with the wet warmth of your tongue and soft moist skin of your lips. Run your tongue languidly around the finger and then suck gently on its tip. Take your time as if you are savouring the very taste of it. Drive her wild!

2. Nibble her fingers and the outer side of her hand teasingly with your teeth. Now take her hand and run it gently over your own face for mutual erotic touching. Let her palm absorb the warmth of your face and her fingers brush across your lips.

3. Rest her hand over her belly so that her fingers settle lightly onto her pubic area. Blow gently onto her hand and then cover it with delicate kisses.

THE BREASTS AND CHEST

Breasts, and in particular nipples, are a highly erogenous zone in both men and women. The many sensitive nerve endings in the nipples and areola (the dark-pigmented skin encircling the nipples) radiate powerful sensations to the emotional and sexual centres of the brain when stimulated by touch, kissing, nuzzling, licking and sucking. This is particularly true for women, whose nipples visibly swell and become erect when sexually excited. Women's breasts, which are composed of milk-secreting glands and fatty tissue, represent an essential part of their femininity and should be touched with a loving respect and awareness even in the most sexually arousing situations. No hard pressure should be applied while massaging the breasts. Before focusing on the breasts erotically, use sensual strokes over the whole of the chest area. Be sure to massage the pectoral muscles above the breasts to ease away tension, allowing your partner's breath and feelings to expand, and enabling her to become more vulnerable and responsive to your touch. Sensual strokes on the face, head and neck (see page 81, The Face) are a wonderful way to follow up the erotic chest and breast massage.

1. Use some pillows or cushions to support your own position as you sit or kneel behind your partner's head. Bring her arms up to lie beside you so that after you stroke up the sides of her ribcage you can slide your hands over her armpits and underarms. Spread oil over the ribcage and onto the arms.

2. Begin the massage with a gentle hold. Place your hands, one softly on top of the other, over her heart area. Let your hands listen to her heart beat, and feel the rise and fall of her breath. See if you can synchronize your own breath into the same undulating rhythm.

3. The first, large movement will be a long, flowing stroke to embrace the whole circumference of her chest. Although there are several stages to the sequence, it should be performed in one unbroken motion and repeated several times.

3 i). Place both hands close together and flat on the top of her chest, with your fingers pointing down her body.

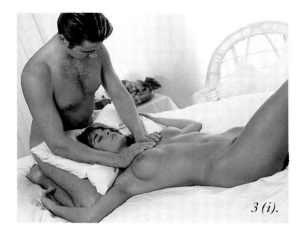

3 (i).

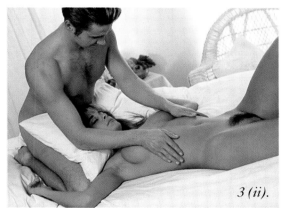

3 (ii).

3 ii). Slide them down her breastbone, and then fan out over the base of her ribcage to the sides of her body.

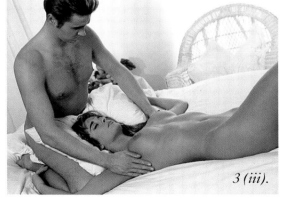

3 (iii).

3 iii). Continue by gliding up the sides of her ribcage, in over her armpits and on to the soft skin of her underarms towards her elbows.

3 iv). Swivel your wrists so your hands can stroke down her arms and onto the pectoral muscles above her breasts. Repeat the sequence.

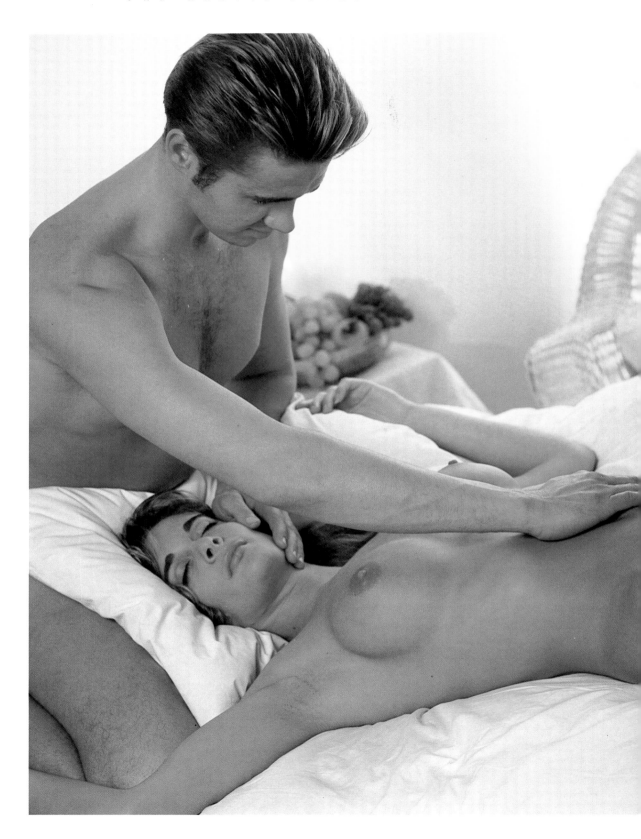

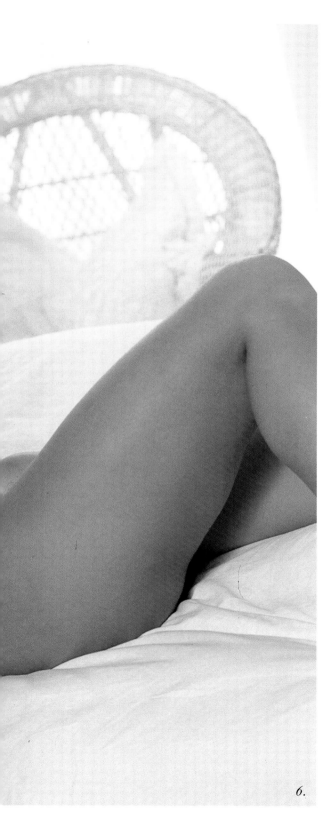

6.

4 i). Place your left hand over your right hand on the base of her breastbone. Draw your hands slowly and steadily up her breastbone with a firm rocking motion which vibrates her ribcage and sends a wave of movement over her heart.

4 ii). At the top of her chest, take away the weight of your left hand and lift your right palm off her body so slowly that the pressure falls through to the fingertips. Lightly trail the fingertips of both hands out over the top of her chest and onto her arms.

5. Glide down her breastbone with both hands, fanning out to the edges of her body. Use the flat of both hands to massage up the sides of her ribcage in spiralling circles while your fingers wrap under and simultaneously stroke her back. Sweep the stroke out over her armpits and arms.

6. Rest your left hand gently on her shoulder while your right hand makes flowing circular movements down her breastbone and on to the soft skin of her belly for as far as you can comfortably reach. This will heighten her anticipation as your downward movements send vibrations through the lower half of her body.

7. Set the skin tingling with tiny feather touches moving up over her chest, breasts and sides of her body and onto her arms. Let the strokes be as light as your partner can bear.

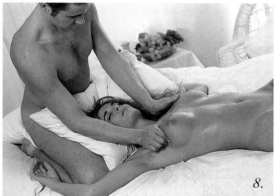

8.

8. Increase pressure on her body again by kneading over her pectoral muscles. Press your fingertips gently into both armpits to anchor your strokes. With one hand alternating with the other on opposite sides of her body, place pressure in your heels and sides of thumbs to roll the muscle towards your fingers. Squeeze and release the flesh as the other hand moves into action.

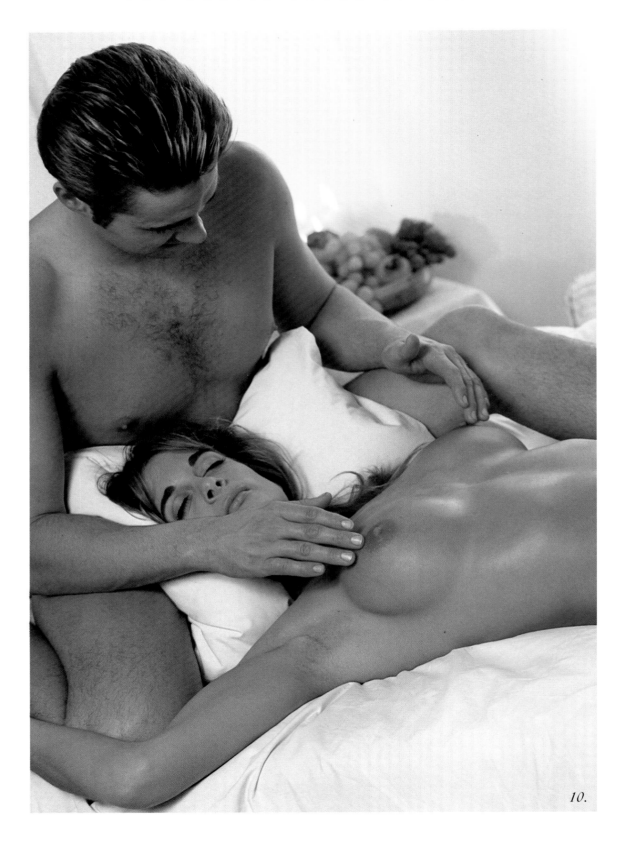

10.

9. To increase the eroticism, cup your hands softly over her breasts, using your fingertips to lightly stroke in decreasing circles towards the nipples, Linger on the areola.

10. Wet both middle fingers with your tongue and delicately rub the moistness over her nipples. You will know if your touch is driving her wild if her nipples swell and her breath deepens.

11. Lovingly diffuse the rising sexual energy so it radiates through her body. Slowly circle your fingers back out over her breasts until your hands reach the sides of her chest. Glide immediately into a full-flowing chest stroke, repeating it several times with varying degrees of pressure and speed, starting with a more vital motion and finishing with a soft, slow touch.

MASSAGING TOWARDS THE BREASTS

If you are kneeling astride your partner's thighs and massaging towards her breasts, adapt the full chest stroke shown in The Chest and Arms (page 78).

1. From this position you can comfortably lean over

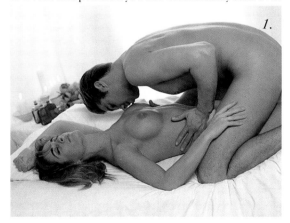

her body to nuzzle, kiss and lick the breasts and nipples with infinite tenderness. However aroused you may become by this intimate contact with her breasts, stay constantly in tune with your partner's responses. Be alert to the signals she is giving through her breathing, sounds and body movement. Let her feel that you respect her body and her sexuality. Again, just bring her to the very edge of excitement before spreading your attention and strokes to the rest of her body in order to infuse her throughout with a constant stream of sexual pleasure.

THE BELLY

Once the abdomen is relaxed by massage, everything about it is sensual. Unprotected by bone, it is soft and round and feels vulnerable to the touch. The belly is a sensitive area where deep emotions and sexual feelings are held and its close proximity to the genitals means that every subtle contact will arouse erotic anticipation.

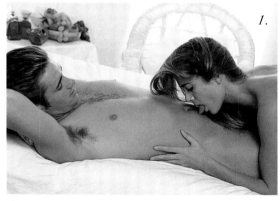

1. Kneeling between your partner's legs, lean over to bring your face close to his belly. Embrace the sides of his body with your hands. Run the tip of your tongue around and around his navel.

2. Rub your face gently over the surface of his belly, brushing its skin with your cheeks, lips and hair.

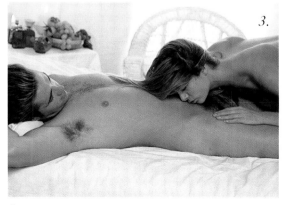

3. Lightly kiss over his entire belly, beginning from just below the ribcage and finishing teasingly just above the pubic bone. If your partner becomes aroused, you can spread those tiny kisses gently over his penis and all around the pubic area. Then move your lips away to kiss softly back over the belly to just below the ribcage, where you began this sensual movement.

THIGHS AND GENITAL AREA

The pubic hair of both men and women serves not only to protect the genital organs from the effects of rubbing together during the act of sex but is also supplied at the roots with some of the most highly erotogenic nerve endings in the body. The arousal response when the hairs are gently pulled, tugged and stroked is stronger in women than in men. Blend your massage on this intensely intimate area with caresses over the belly and thighs.

1. Massage and relax your partner's legs and feet. Ease open her groin and genital area by resting her lower leg on your shoulder so that her knee is flexed. Stroke several times up both sides of her thigh with your hands, gliding them back down behind her leg. Use the hand closest to her body or the soft skin of your forearm to circle-stroke up and down her inner thigh. Rest her leg back on the mattress and apply the same attention to the other side of her body.

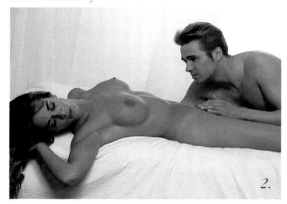

2. Kneel between her knees to lean over and cover her belly with kisses from your lips and tongue. Having awakened the whole area surrounding her genitals, gently stroke around her mons veneris, the padded area of the public bone. Teasingly tug on the pubic hair and comb your fingertips through it. Never rush or be intrusive with your strokes when massaging the genital area. While your lover may become aroused, your touch should convey how deeply you treasure this access to her most intimate parts. Your fingertips should speak of the wonder you feel in being able to caress her secret pleasure zones. Allow your sexual desire to be there but do not impose it upon her. Let it ripen slowly like a fruit in season.

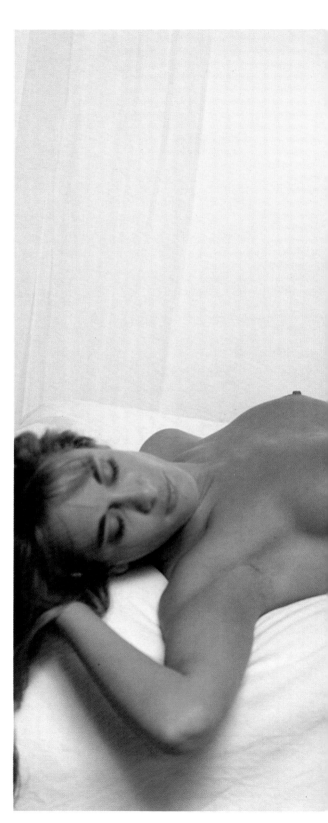

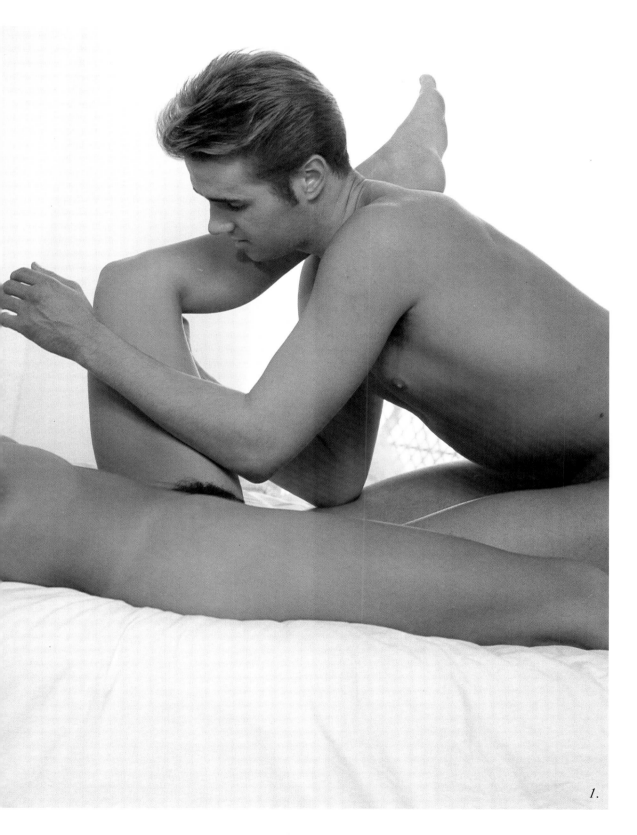

1.

THE PENIS AND SCROTUM

Too much activity focused on the penis will send your man into a state of excitement, and you may have to abandon the massage! Continued stimulation of the penis will almost certainly bring him to orgasm. Honour the penis and scrotum with your loving touches, yet take care to diffuse the stimulation by spreading your strokes over the rest of his body. Remember to keep the temperature on the boil, but not boiling over! The penis is the most sexually responsive part of a man's body, with thousands of highly sensitive nerve endings lining its soft, sensitive skin. The scrotum is the sac beneath the penis containing the two testicles, the male sex glands. Stroking the scrotum will also produce very pleasurable and sexually-charged sensations for your partner, but be very tender – this is a fragile area.

1. Use your sensual stretch strokes to massage all over his thighs and belly, sweeping your hand over his penis as it lies on his thigh. Gently caress the scrotum and penis as your hands free-flow.

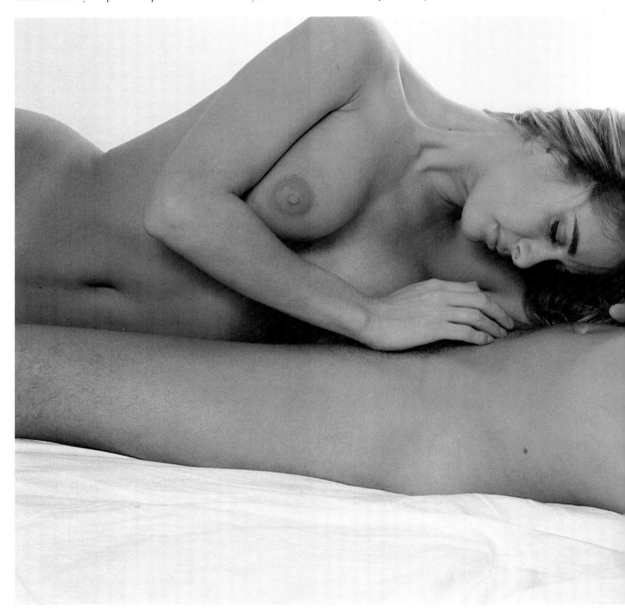

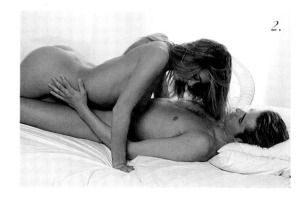

2.

2. As the penis swells and becomes more erect, clasp it in one hand and stroke down its shaft, from the tip to its base. Loosen your hold slightly as your hand glides back. Repeat several times, while fondling the scrotum with your other hand. Cover the penis with delicate kisses and soft brushes of your lips.

3. Move your hand away from his penis before it becomes fully erect. Support your weight with your hands, and sensually slide your breasts over his genitals.

1.

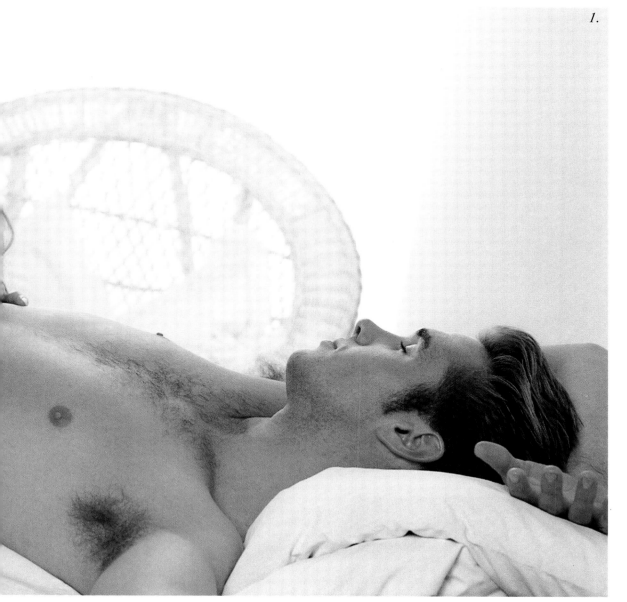

1.

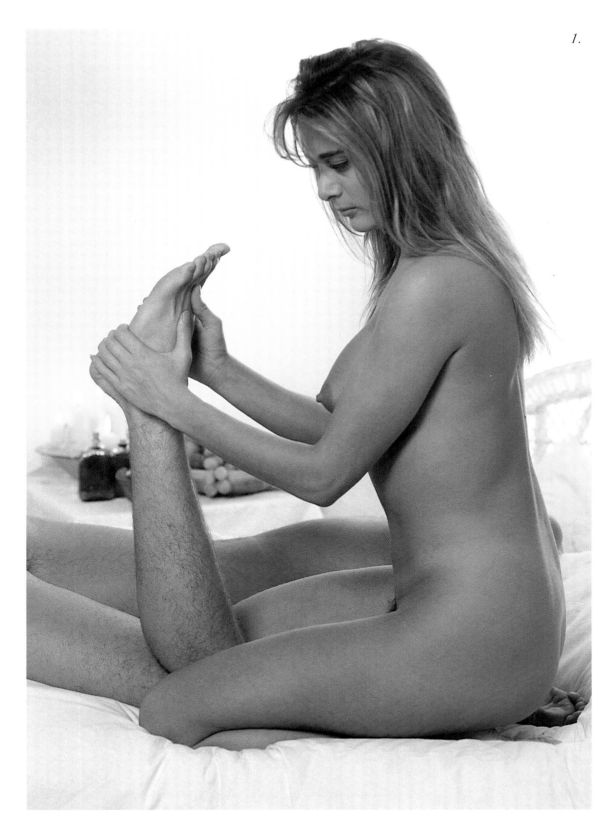

FEET AND TOES

To create a more sensuous and erotic foot massage, bring your partner's foot into closer contact with your own body. From this position you can massage, kiss, lick and blow over his toes to send a stream of sensation sizzling through the whole nervous system.

1. Raise his lower leg so it is supported by the knee and rest it against the soft curve of your breast and shoulder. Clasp his foot so that your fingers rest across the sole and your thumbs over the instep. Fan one thumb after the other in firm circular motions, emphasizing pressure on the outward sweep and gliding back around lightly. Let your fingers simultaneously stroke over the sole. Work over the instep to the base of the toes, slipping your hands back down and around his ankles to repeat the sequence. Adapt the foot massage strokes to this new position.

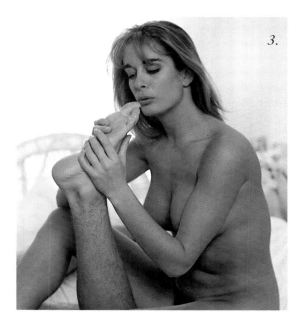

3.

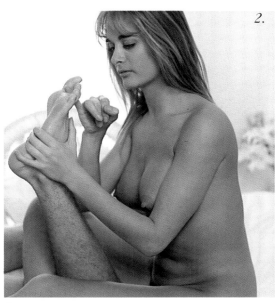

2.

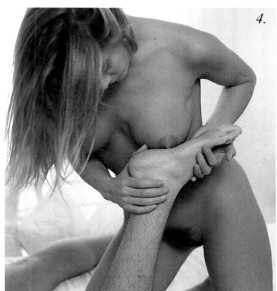

4.

2. Friction on the delicate skin between the toes feels amazingly sensual. Slide your index finger between each toe and twist it back and forth in a cork screw motion.

3. Toes are famous for being sexy and responsive to erotic sensation. Begin by blowing softly all over his foot. Using the gentlest of pressure, playfully bite and suck on the ends of his toes. Pay special attention to his big toe. Dry the moistness from the toes with the heat of your breath.

4. Take his foot and fondle it against your breasts. Brush the sole with a delicate sweep of your nipple. Then slide his foot and lower leg against your body, massaging it with your chest and belly as you twist sensually from side to side.

5. Place the foot back on the mattress so that it rests between your legs. Supporting your weight, lower your body so that you gently press onto the foot with your genital area for several moments, then slowly release the pressure. Your partner will long to receive the same attention on his other foot.

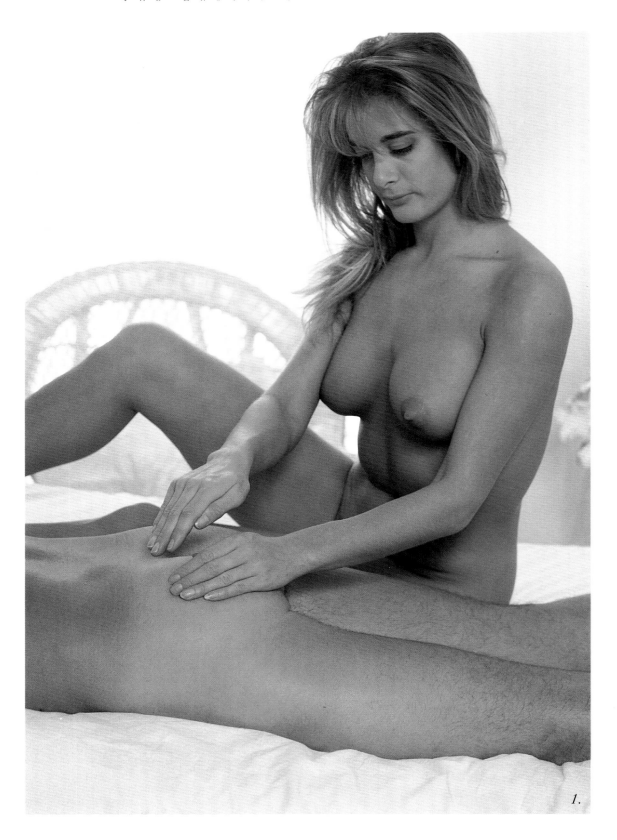

1.

THE BUTTOCKS

While most of the sequences described in this chapter have involved soft, tender touches and cherishing caresses, you can add some vigorous movements to your erotic massage for a touch of spice and vitality! The best place to apply them is over the back of the thighs and buttocks. Men seem to particularly enjoy these stimulating strokes on the cheeks of their buttocks.

1. Stroke over your partner's thighs and buttocks with the flat of your hands so that they mould into the curvaceous shapes. Then work thoroughly over the fleshy areas with the strong kneading strokes described in Sexual Tension in the Buttocks (page 44).

2. Kneel or sit by your partner's hip and apply a series of percussion strokes. Start with hacking, (How It Works, page 17), and strike briskly over his buttocks and tops of his legs so the blood circulation is boosted to the surface of the skin.

3. Cup your hands to create a vacuum in the centre of your palms. Your fingers should be straight and close together with your thumbs drawn in. Keeping your wrists loose, strike the skin with both hands moving in quick succession, flicking them back off the body as soon as they make contact. This cupping stroke should produce a muted, naughty-but-nice slapping sound! Now tease the skin with feather touches.

THE BACK, NECK AND EARS

Most people know the thrill of a lover's kisses caressing the neck and ears. Bring an erotic play of lips and tongue into your massage as you stroke over your partner's back, neck and ears.

1. Kneeling astride your partner's thighs, stroke sensually over her back. Slither around over her body so that she feels the the gentle sweep of your genitals against her buttocks, and the heat of your belly and chest above her skin.

2. To send exciting shivers up and down her spine, run the tip of your tongue swiftly up along its vertebrae from the base by the fold of the buttocks right up to the very top of her neck. Repeat the movement up the spine with your tongue, but this time flicking it slightly from side to side over each vertebra.

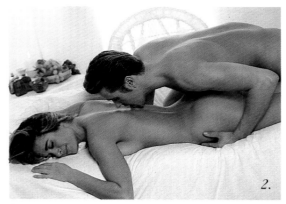

2.

3. Slide off her body, and whisper to your partner to curl up onto her side so that she faces away from you. Stroke caringly through her hair to brush it away from her neck and ears.

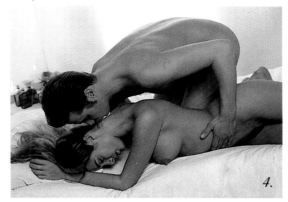

4.

4. Draw her close to you and, leaning over her comfortably, plant distinct but tiny kisses over her neck and along her hair line.

5. Move your lips to her ear, kissing and nibbling over the lobe and rim. Let the tip of your tongue seductively trace over the ear's intricate shape. As her body surrenders, lovingly stroke over her breasts and belly.

THE PRELUDE TO MAKING LOVE

Your erotic massage has been a sumptuous occasion of body worship, dissolving the boundary between sensuality and sexuality. Every inch of skin on your partner's body has been loved and cherished. With the senses alive and every cell expectant and throbbing, undoubtedly you both will be ready to make love. What follows next could be the most exquisite stage in your exploration and experience of the phenomenon of loving touch.

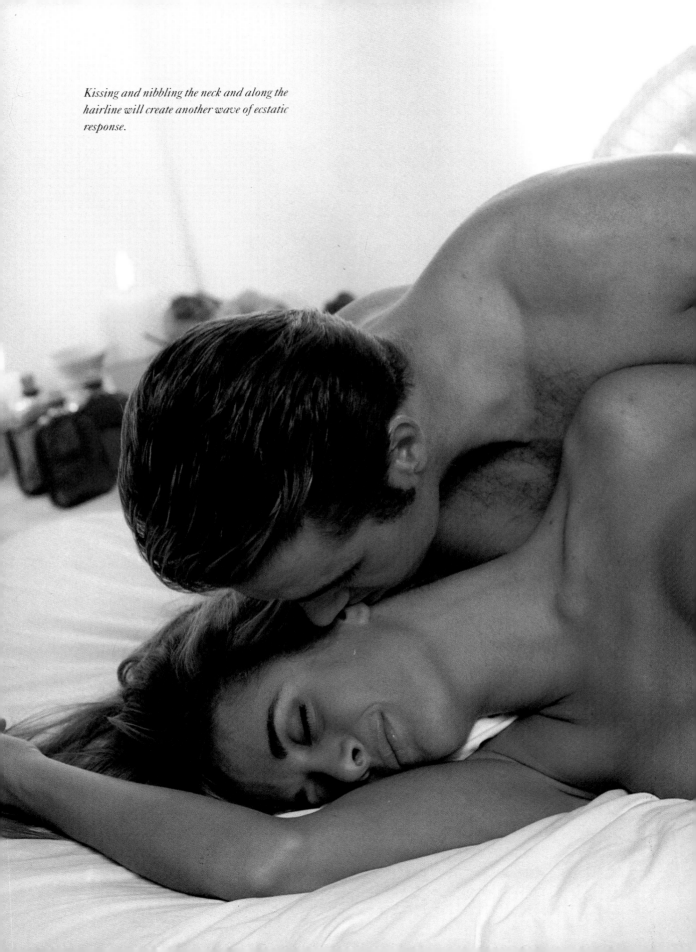

Kissing and nibbling the neck and along the hairline will create another wave of ecstatic response.

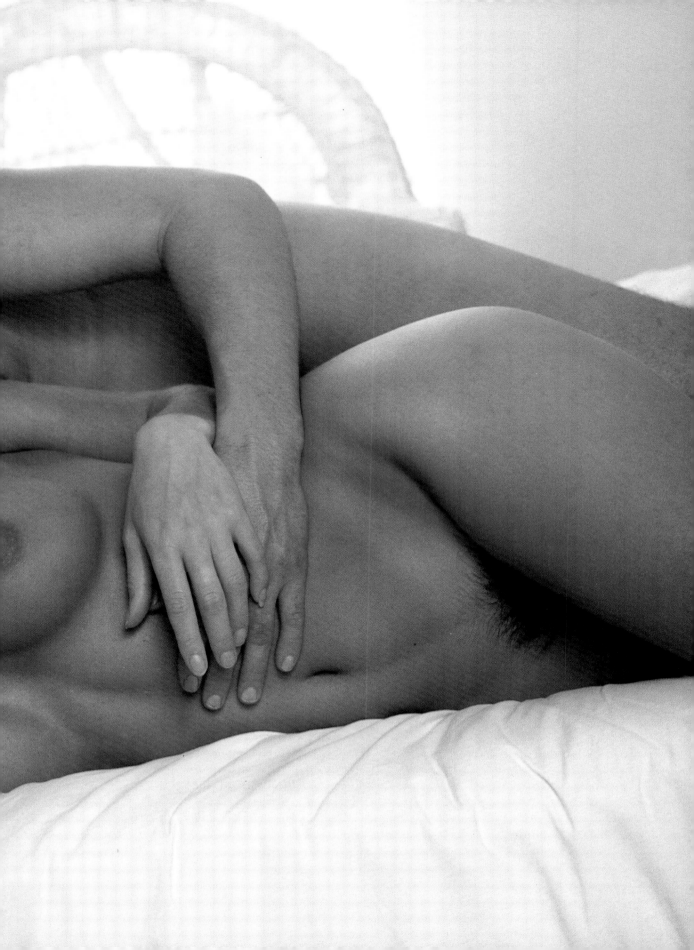

Entering the temple of the spirit

By bringing your sensual and erotic massage techniques into the sexual experience,

you can stay in tune with your lover during those special moments of deep intimacy.

For while sensuality can exist without sexuality, sex is always richer

for the inclusion of a continuing sensitivity and appreciation of the whole

body through loving touch.

AT THE HEIGHT of the sexual act, as penetration occurs and the partners move into different sexual positions, the joy of tactile communication should remain integral to making love. This may require developing a slower, more sensitive and aware approach to making love, especially if you have previously thought of foreplay and sensuality only as a prelude to the 'real thing' – achieving enough excitement to rush headlong towards a successful orgasm. Ask yourself how often, while making love, you have secretly felt that you have lost your lover somewhere along the way in the race towards the finishing line.

While making love, it is easy to lose the intimate connection with your partner in the course of your own excitement and fantasy. Private sexual fantasies can overtake the mind, so that sex becomes an almost cerebral affair, and frenzied activity occurs in order to stimulate the sexual organs to reach a physical climax. Tension builds up in the body and mind to be subsequently released during

Loving touch should always be a part of sexual union.

108

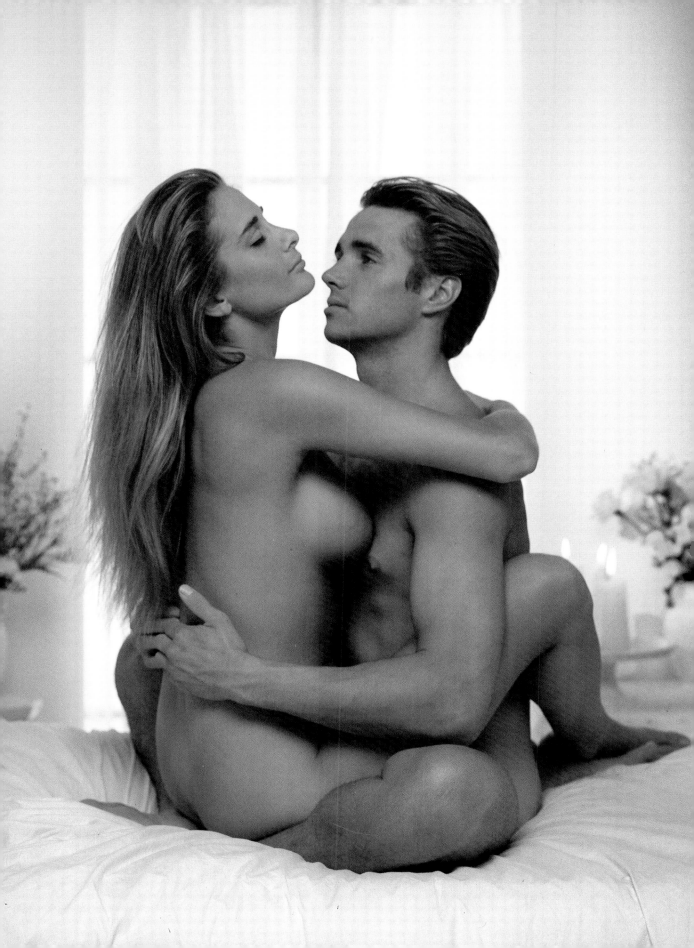

the involuntary contractions of pelvic floor muscles, creating the wave-like and pleasurable sensations of orgasm.

While fantasy and physical technique can be used to achieve the desired goal of orgasm, they can result in the couple missing the emotional vulnerability and love that should surely exist between them in these moments of deepest union. Men frequently feel depleted of energy after ejaculation, needing to cut off temporarily from their partners or go to sleep. Women tend to become more energized after orgasm, and often feel abandoned and dissatisfied at the very moment when they most desire intimacy. In fact, a high proportion of women do not achieve orgasm at all during the sexual act, often needing more time to relax and feel cherished.

Both partners may worry unduly about the 'orgasm factor', and this very concern spoils the spontaneous expression of love and harmonious union that is possible during intercourse. A man may feel anxious about ejaculating before he is able to satisfy his partner, so he sets about trying to arouse the woman as if she were a machine rather than a human being. He may start to memorize figures or think about his favourite football team in an effort to delay his orgasm. While he has his woman in his arms, he is a million miles away from her. His partner, on the other hand, may be frantically trying to conjure up sexual imagery to increase her arousal either to achieve an orgasm before her man climaxes, or because she feels that it is her duty to have one. She may fake an orgasm to soothe his ego, or, conversely, blame him for not satisfying her. When they have completed their sexual act, the two people involved may feel more distant from each other than when they first started.

While orgasm is a definite fulfilment in intercourse, it is only one dimension of the act of making love. Instead of pursuing orgasm as the only goal, the message in this chapter is to slow down, breathe deeply together, make more eye-contact, move slowly together, be playful and continue to touch and massage not only the obvious erogenous zones but every part of your partner's body. Then, instead of twiddling with and rubbing parts of the body in order to reach an end result, your love-making can

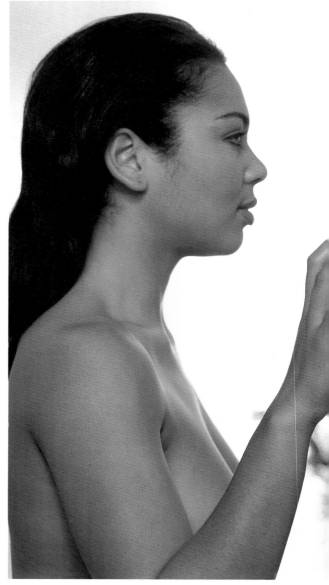

move into another realm altogether. Let the waves of sexual and orgasmic pleasure spread from the pelvic area through the whole body, coursing through the cells to skin level in response to your loving caresses. Forget for a while the big 'O' and relax into the pleasure of communicating to every part of the body with each touch and stroke, not only your sexual desire for each other but also a sense of deep appreciation for the whole person with whom you are sharing this special moment.

While you may at first be self-conscious about changing the pattern of your love-making, with

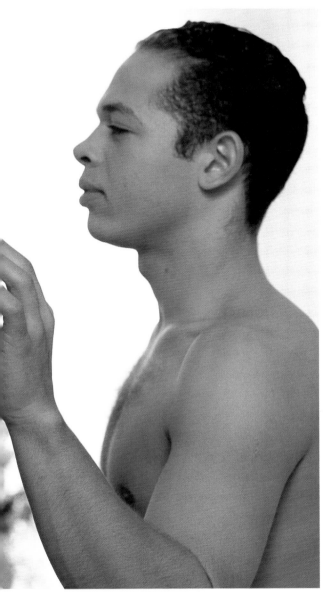

When sexual arousal is kindled, the fingertips become highly sensitive and erotogenic. Feel the pulsation pass between you by bringing the fingertips together.

mutual willingness and trust in the exploration you will both experience its rewards. By staying constantly in the moment and continuously relating to each other, by allowing yourselves to relax instead of becoming tense with sexual excitement, you can ride along the waves of joyful sexual energy. Signal to each other to slow down in movement if either of you is becoming too excited. When you reach a peak of excitement and before you lose control, become still. Consciously let your breathing grow slower and deeper, allowing the orgasmic sensations to spread away from the genital area with the gentle caress and massage of your hands over your partner's body.

Let your bodies melt into an embrace, synchronizing the inhalation and exhalation of your breath so that you become united almost as one energy. Move the pelvis gently when necessary to maintain the erection of the penis inside the vagina, taking care not to overstimulate the sexual organs into orgasm before you are ready. The woman can contract her vaginal muscles to clasp and release the penis to keep it erect. Lying still, touching each other and breathing together allows a whole wave of sexual energy to emerge naturally on its own without mental interference. Let it build up slowly until it takes over and moves you into active lovemaking again. In this way, you can continue your loving for luxuriously long periods of time because you are not programming yourselves towards an end result or depleting yourselves prematurely through climax and ejaculation.

THE SACREDNESS OF SEX

In ancient Eastern philosophies there was a profound understanding of the sacredness of sex. The Taoist philosophy taught people to live in harmony with the unchanging laws of nature, born from the equilibrium of heaven and earth and governed by the merging of the bright, active male yang energy of the Sky with the dark, passive and intuitive female yin energy of the Earth. The ancient Taoist symbol of Yin -Yang, with its black and white curled motifs entwined within a circle, each carrying a dot of the opposing colour, has now become a popular emblem for universal harmony in the Western world. The Chinese teachers of Tao did not believe in separating earthly and heavenly pleasures but encouraged a conscious experience of both. They believed the sexual union of man and woman was a microcosm of the greater cosmic law. Not only did it benefit the health and wellbeing of men and women, but with the right practice it empowered their spiritual lives. They strongly advocated control of ejaculation so that a man could fully satisfy his woman, prolong his love-making, and at the same time preserve his vital life-force. To this end, many texts were written on the art of sex which were poetic in language but contained a sound medical and scientific basis.

The Tantric masters of India and Tibet also believed in universal harmony based on the inter-action and unity of the cosmic forces of male and female energy. For many thousands of years, Hindus have worshipped at the shrines of the god Shiva and his consort Shakti, personified by the lingam and yoni, stone sculptures of the united penis and vagina. Hindu Tantra taught that sex was a path to super-consciousness, the ultimate state of spiritual enlightenment and truth. Initiates into Tantra learnt yogic sexual practices, combining sexual positions with breathing techniques to awaken the spiritual energy centres contained within the human body. According to the Tantric masters, this vibrational flow of the vital life force, known as kundalini, originates in the sex centre at the base of the spine. On release, it streams its way up through the energy centres of the body, known as chakras, towards the crown of the head, transforming ordinary consciousness into one of awakened ecstasy. Tantric sexual practices teach that the body is the tabernacle of love within which reside the divine qualities of each man and woman and that love-making should ultimately acknowledge the god and goddess within. The mystics of ancient Egypt and Greece also exalted the sex act as representative of the eternal and universal processes of life, death and regeneration.

Today, both Tantric and Taoist teachings are gaining popularity amongst Western people who seek to bring a spiritual and ecstatic quality into their lives. Many books are now available which translate the ancient teachings into modern terms so that their practices have more relevance to the West.

Allow stillness and calm to become part of your lovemaking so that it has the quality of meditation. Let your bodies merge as one.

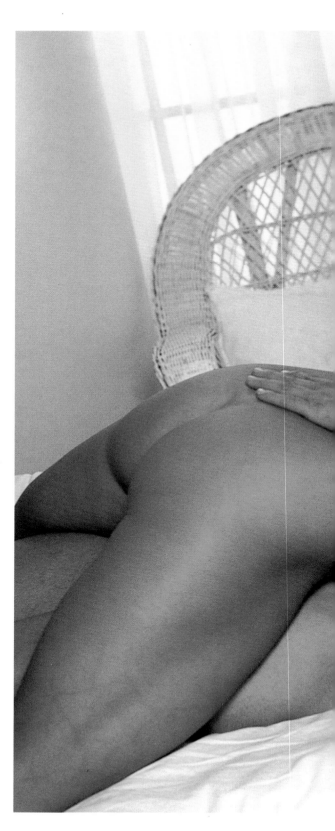

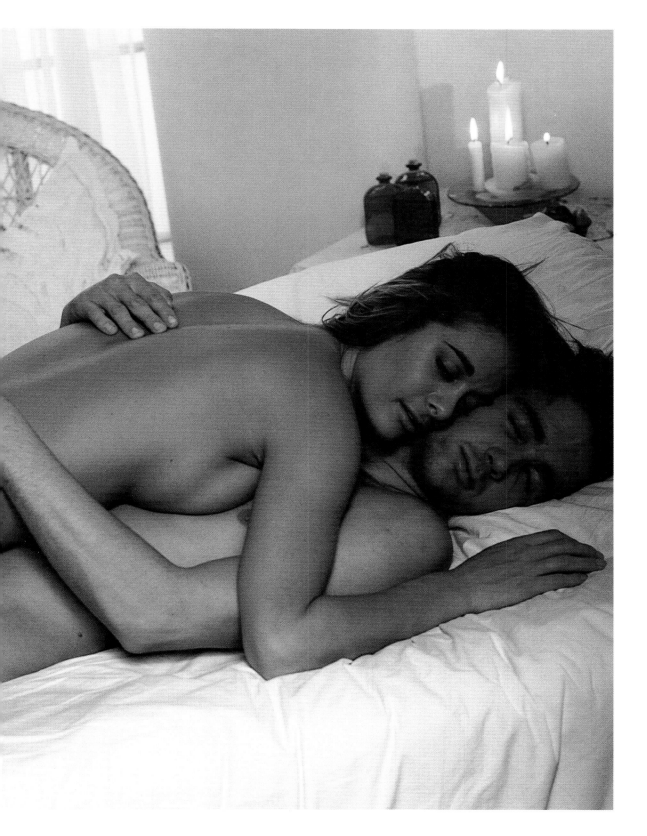

MASSAGE AS A MEDIUM OF LOVE

If you and your partner have been following the massage sequences presented in previous chapters, you will know by now just how alive and relaxed you can become through giving and receiving massage. The close association between touch, skin and feelings will also have become obvious to you. In fact, our language shows that we have an instinctive understanding of how these three aspects of our body and being are enmeshed. We substitute the word feel for touch, when, for example, we invite someone to feel the luxurious quality of a silken texture. We say we are touched when warm and vulnerable feelings are evoked. Expressions such as "skin deep", or "I've got you under my skin", suggest an emotional response with its base in physicality.

You will have discovered how massage and loving touch enable you to penetrate the physical and psychological barriers of the body and mind to bring you into intimate contact with the essential being of the person you love. In this way, massage has an almost transcendental quality. It is like making love and has an orgasmic energy of its own. Correctly practised, it can become a meditation and an act of love. If you begin to view sex as a sacred act, touch as a medium of love, and your own body and that of your lover as temples of worship, then massage and making love can combine perfectly to bring a more profound dimension into intimacy.

Let massage and touch continue to function as a part of your love-making, not only as an enhancement to relaxation, sensuality and eroticism, but also as an integral spiritual part of your loving sexual act.

The following programmes are offered only as suggestions with which you and your lover may wish to experiment. Use or adapt them in any way that will enhance your sexual relationship.

EXERCISE IN INCREASING TOUCH AWARENESS

If you do not have the time to give a full body massage to your lover but wish to create a mood of physical intimacy and heighten the senses before making love, this exercise is a playful way to increase skin awareness and the sense of touch.

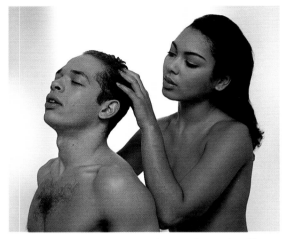

Even a quick massage, such as here on the head, will start the process of physical bonding so necessary if you are to be available and open to each other sexually.

The key to the first part of this exercise lies in introducing a playful element of surprise to tactile contact so as to increase the receiver's anticipation of touch. By sitting passively with closed eyes, or even blindfolded lightly by a silk scarf, your partner will be unable to tell from which direction your touch will come, or where it will settle on the body. The dominating sense of vision is therefore sublimated to the skin's nerve network, causing the skin to become alive with expectation. Where you touch and how you touch will vary, but your hands should always be sensitive, settling on the body with the lightness of a leaf carried by a breeze to the earth. Wherever they rest, bring all your attention into your hands and the underlying body area so that every touch resonates with your presence, vitality and awareness.

Close your eyes and let your hands 'listen' to the body's internal music: the beating of the heart, the throb of the pulse, the rhythm of the breath. Move quietly around your partner. Always take time between each contact to withdraw so as to increase the anticipation of your touch.

1. If you are behind your partner, you may want to place one hand softly onto her brow and the other over her heart. After some moments of repose, withdraw your hands just as delicately and then place them on another area such as the shoulders.

1.

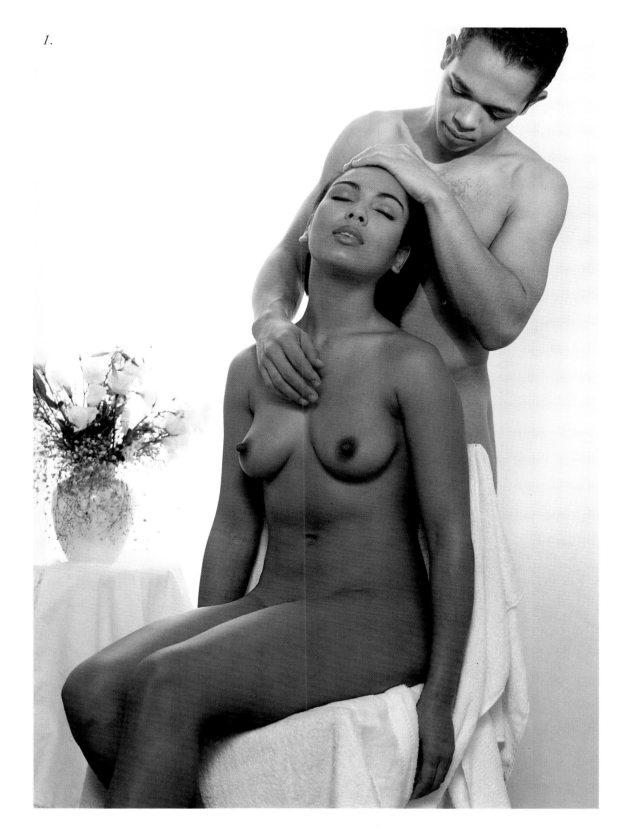

Move silently to her side, letting one hand cup the nape of her neck while the other settles on her belly. Come in front of your partner and rest your hands gently over her breasts, thighs, knees or feet.

2.   Let your touches be sensual and teasing. Continuing to move around her, stroke her hair, caress her face, brush her nipples with your breath or feather along the soft surface of the inner thighs with your fingertips.

3.   Now let your touch be more intuitive so that your hands float to areas of the body of their own free will without being directed by your mind. If you give yourself permission to trust your hands' innate responses you will be surprised how they

4.

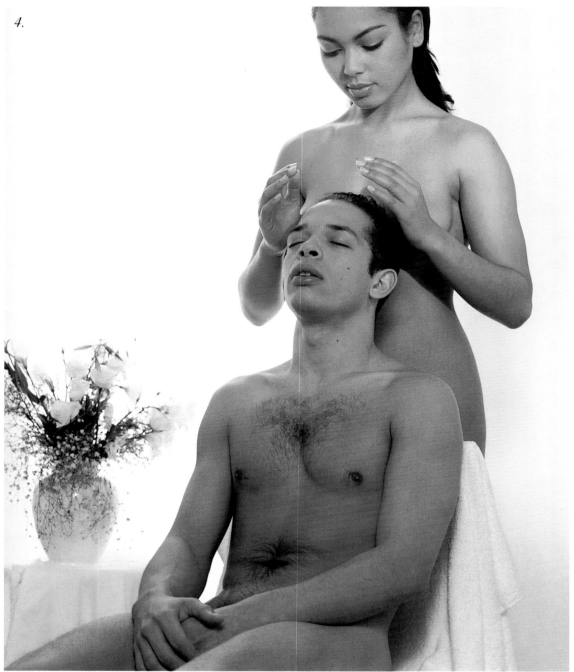

seem to have a movement and feeling sense of their own. Close your eyes, tune in to your partner through touch and see if his body, mind or emotions have a message for you.

4. The idea that an energy field surrounds the human body is one that has been long accepted by psychics, healers and mystics. The more sensitive your hands become to the whole person through massage, the more likely it is that they will begin to feel the subtle sense of light, heat and vibration emanating from the body. Explore this potential with your partner, approaching the body slowly and sensitively but keeping your hands a few inches away from its surface. Focus on key energy spots, such as the abdomen, solar plexus, heart, spine and crown of the head. Even though your hands are off the body, they will have a deep sense of connection to your partner just as he will be aware of their presence and vitality. Always withdraw your hands slowly out of the 'energy field' before moving to another area.

BONDING THROUGH EYE CONTACT, BREATH AND TOUCH

Beneath the outer self that we present to the world we all have a vulnerable side to our nature. Yet because this feels fragile and childlike, we try hard not to reveal it to other people. Under the spotlight of everyday life, it usually makes sense to guard these tender emotions. However, real intimacy with a partner builds trust so that we can feel safe to share our innermost feelings – and love is the most vulnerable feeling of all.

This exercise uses eye contact, breath and calm gentle touch to help you bond and share emotionally while making love. The woman should sit astride her partner, moving the pelvis or tightening her vagina only enough to help him maintain his erection. To go fully into this exercise, relax into the waves of sexual pleasure but avoid becoming overstimulated.

1. The eyes are said to be the mirrors of the soul. To look deeply into each other's eyes is to be willing to expose our inner truth. Hold each other gently, but in such a way that it is easy to maintain maximum eye-contact. Do not try to out-stare each other. Your eyes should be softly focused and

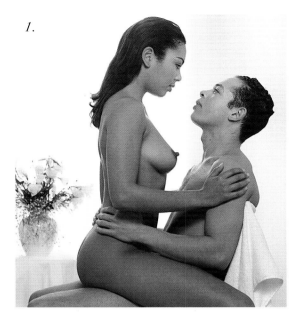

1.

receptive as if to allow your partner into the secrets of your heart. Let your thoughts and feelings come and go without trying to control them, and allow your breathing to wash away any tensions which arise. Relax your face and body whenever they tighten up. Keep breathing and looking into each other's eyes until all barriers have dissolved.

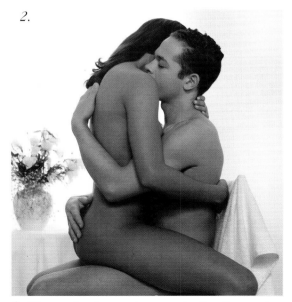

2.

2. Hug each other so that your bodies fit together and close your eyes. Feel every inch of the skin-to-skin contact this position gives you. Tune in to your own breathing and witness the rise and fall of your breath as it moves through you. After a while, begin to focus on the rhythm of your partner's breathing, noticing the expansion of the chest and belly against your own on inhalation and the contraction on exhalation. Gradually begin to synchronize your breathing patterns, taking the breath in through your nose and letting it sink down into your genitals. Breathe out as if from your genitals, expelling the breath through your entire body. Keep breathing together in this way until you both feel you are one body and one flow of breath. Slowly, you should begin to experience a build-up of warmth and vibration within the genital area. Remain relaxed and allow these sensations to pulsate within you without moving into action.

3.

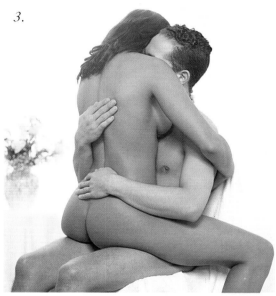

3. As the male partner, you are now in a position to make a series of tender holds to guide the releasing sexual energy up through your lover's body and along her spine. Focus your attention into your hands while she directs her breath to meet your touch. Keep your right hand over the sacrum at the base of the spine and lay the other hand slightly above it. After some moments move your left hand to rest on the centre of her spine, behind the solar plexus. Next, put your left hand on the part of the spine that is in proximity to her heart. Now move your arm upwards so that your hand covers the nape of her neck. Finally, place your hand tenderly over the crown of her head.

THE KUNDALINI MASSAGE

The kundalini exercises which form part of the yogic tradition of Tantra are usually taught by a Tantric teacher and may involve many months or even years of preparation and practice. They are part of a spiritual way of life and students need guidance through each stage of the energy-transforming meditations.

The massage programme suggested here is named kundalini massage because it helps you to release tensions from the spine while making love so that it becomes flexible and more able to transport the orgasmic waves of pleasure through the entire nervous system. You can begin by adapting and using the previous exercise to increase your emotional and physical openness to one another. The eye-contact, breathing and touch will have helped to dissolve any remaining emotional barriers, enabling the rising sexual energy to infuse your cells.

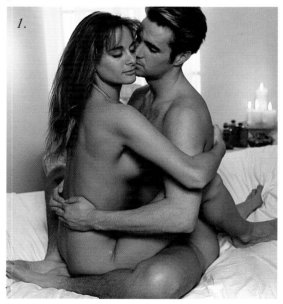

1. If you are making love in a sitting position on the bed or floor, the woman should wrap her legs around her man's pelvis, or place her feet onto the firm surface to give her support. Begin to sway gently as if to uncoil the sexual vibrations and send them spiralling up through your spine. Both partners can massage each other's spines simultaneously or in turn, working the fingertips in tiny rotations on one spot at a time along the edges of the

2.

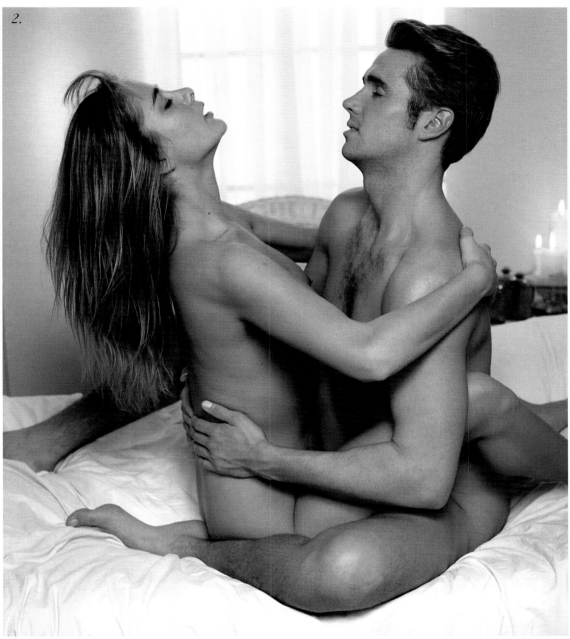

vertebrae from the sacrum to the top of the neck. Give extra attention to any areas that remain tense and unyielding, while your partner directs breath to that part. After massaging the spine, stroke your hands over the scalp and up through the hair as if releasing the rising sensations out through the top of the head.

2. When the whole back and spine is loosened and the sexual energy is reaching a peak, abandon your-selves to the joy of sex. Let your breath take on its own momentum as you sway and vibrate with ecstasy. Remember that all the breathing, move-ment and massage while making love can release some powerful sensations and feelings. You may find yourself making sounds, laughing or perhaps crying. Give yourself permission to express your responses uninhibitedly and you will feel wonder-fully liberated.

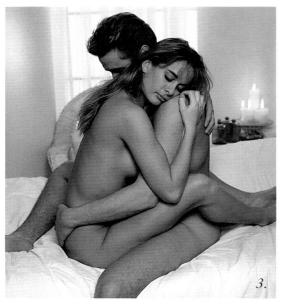

3.

3. If you are moving spontaneously towards orgasm, and if this is what you both desire, let go into the climax. However, if you wish to prolong your love-making and take it into another dimension, let the waves of orgasmic energy roll back into a calm lull before surging towards another crest. Either way, hold each other and stay emotionally and physically connected. Breathe together and feel your hearts beating as the energy subsides. Melt into each other's arms.

CHOOSING POSITIONS TO RELAX AND MAKE LOVE

When your love-making is relaxed, your bodies will move and roll easily from one position to another without the effort of Olympian gymnastics. The ease with which your body flows in this state enables it to feel light and weightless. Your limbs can wrap and unfold with natural grace because you are moving with an inner energy rather than trying to achieve a mind-controlled position. Varying your positions during sex adds variety and spice to your love-making, allowing each partner to take turns in active and passive roles. Some positions are useful to prolong the period before orgasm, while others help to stimulate the sexual organs and speed up the process. It is good for your sex life to be inventive but the important thing is for both partners to be in agreement and to feel comfortable

about any position, so communication is vital.

The positions shown here are to inspire you to continue using massage and loving touch as part of your sexual experience. By allowing you to reach and touch a maximum area of the body, they will keep you focused on the pleasure of whole body and skin stimulation instead of opting only for genital arousal or zoning in exclusively on the most obvious erogenous parts such as the mouth and breasts.

If you massage while making love, you can simply touch the body spontaneously, caressing the skin in tender responses as the mood takes you. Alternatively, keep a bottle or bowl of oil containing erotic essential oils close to your bed for use in the slower and more passive moments of sex to perform appropriate strokes learnt in previous chapters. While making love, let your hands and fingers continue to linger on and caress the face and skin, stroke up the spine, deftly manipulate and knead the buttocks and thighs, massage the chest, breasts and arms, and softly rub the belly. These strokes will continue to add to the sensuality and joy of what is already a wonderful experience.

1. If you have been following the massage sequences you will know by now how sensuous the buttocks are. Most sexual positions allow you easy access to stroke and knead their voluptuous curves. Caressing and gently squeezing the cheeks will heighten passion. In this adventurous sexual position, the woman turns her back to her partner as she straddles over him. While this does not have the intimacy of front-to-front contact, it can be an exciting sexual moment because the buttocks are a visually stimulating and erogenous zone for both sexes. As you move together, heighten the erotic sensitivity of this area by stroking and kneading the strong muscles.

2. One advantage of the woman kneeling astride and facing her partner during penetration is that she is in control of the depth and speed of the thrusts of her partner's penis into her vagina. Many men

The buttocks are a highly erotic zone. Gentle kneading of the muscles while making love will heighten arousal in this adventurous position.

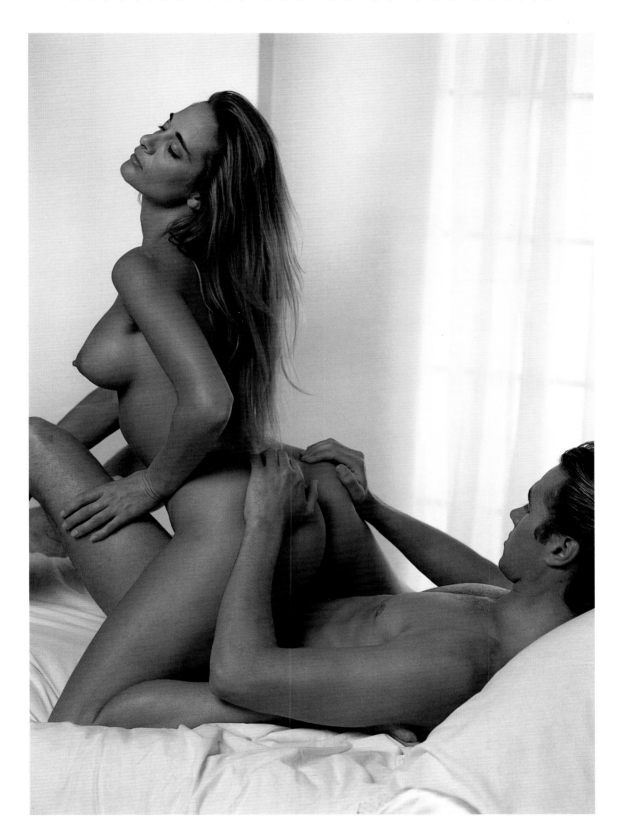

welcome the respite from being the active lover, enjoying the opportunity to lie back and become passive. When it feels right, as the woman, you can slow down the action, moving your pelvis only to help him keep his erection inside of you.

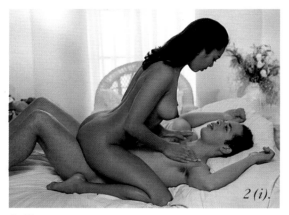

2 (i). From this position, you can easily massage the top of his chest and shoulders. Warm a little oil between your hands and spread it lovingly all over the chest and upper arms. Sweep your hands up over his breastbone, then lean your weight into your hands as they glide out over the pectoral muscles. Take your stroke over the top of his arms, then curve your hands so they slide back down and along the sides of the ribcage before pulling them back in towards the starting place of the first stroke. Repeat this motion several times to bring a vibrancy to his chest.

3. Adapt the face massage strokes to this position, adding whatever loving touches most express your intimate feelings at this moment.

4. At this point both of you may want to return to raising the sexual stakes. Enjoy and let go into love-making, but again slow down before you reach a momentum over which you no longer have control if you wish to return the compliment of massage to your woman.

5. The woman is in the perfect position to arch herself back against the support of your knees, revealing to you the full beauty of her body. Embrace and honour it with your touches. Add a little oil to your hands and stroke over the soft roundness of her belly with circular and fan-shaped motions.

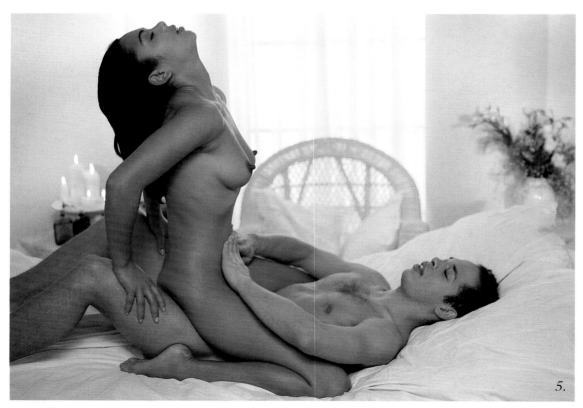

5.

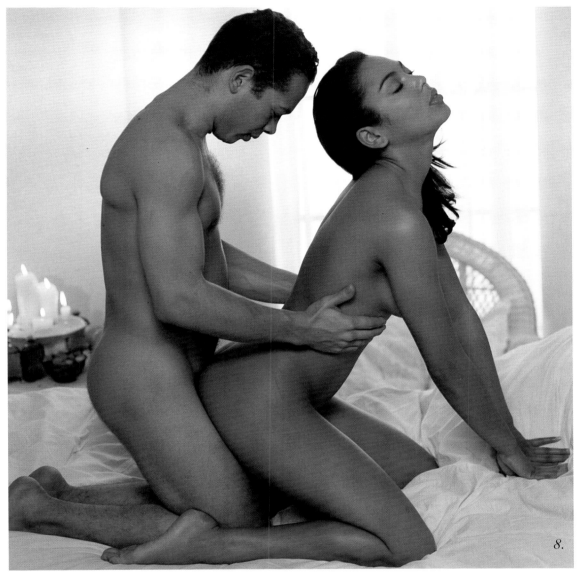

8.

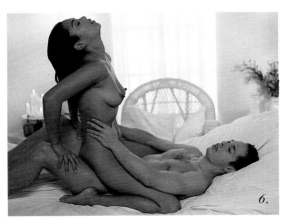

6.

6. Glide your hands up along the sides of her body and around the curvaceous lines of her hips and waist, repeating the motion several times.

7. Now stroke all over her thighs, flexing your wrists to slide your hands along the inner thighs and groin and then to encircle the full pelvic girdle.

8. Entering the vagina from the rear position can be an exciting turn-on for both partners, and it also provides the man with an opportunity of lovingly stroking and caressing the woman's breasts, belly, pubic area and clitoris while making love to her at the same time. Let your strokes be soft and flowing, honouring both her internal and external beauty.

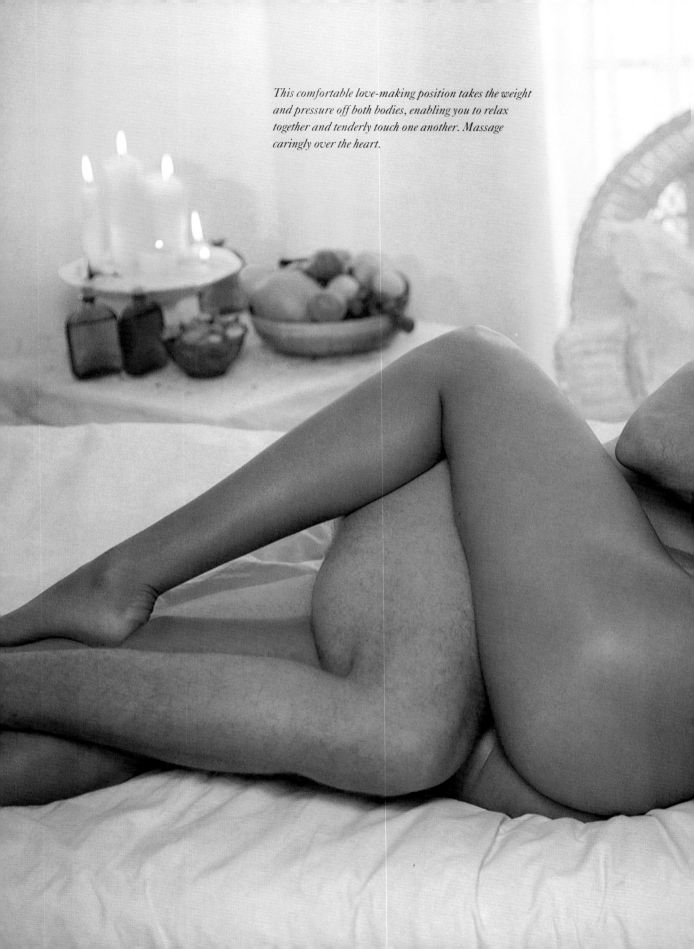

This comfortable love-making position takes the weight and pressure off both bodies, enabling you to relax together and tenderly touch one another. Massage caringly over the heart.

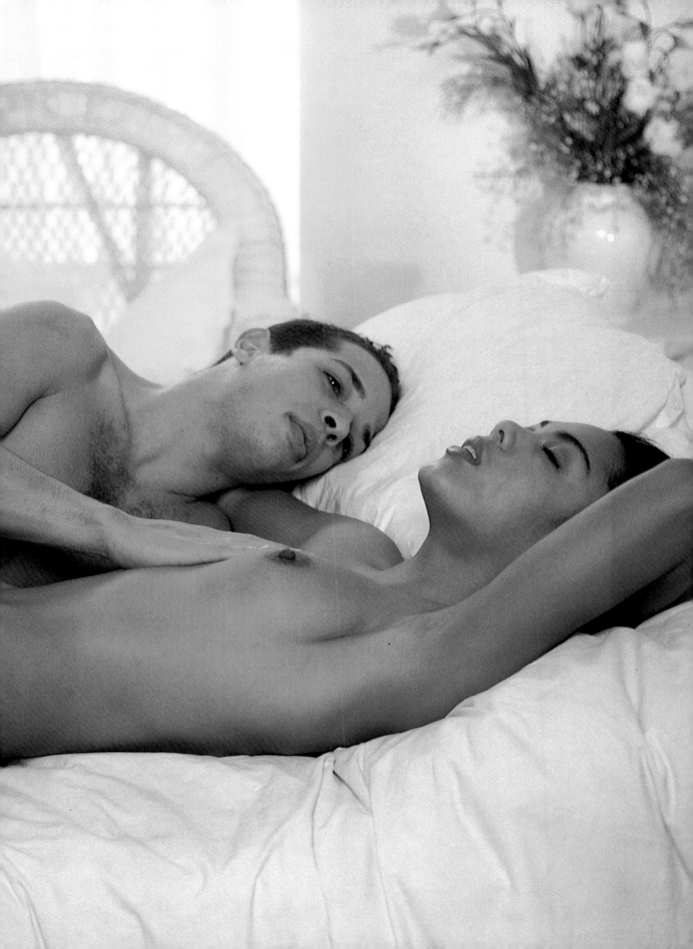

9. When the mood of sex turns into pure tenderness, one of the most relaxed postures to adopt is lying face to face on your side, or in the scissors position shown on the previous page. This leaves the abdomen and back free from pressure and stress. You can exchange loving words and touch and massage each other over many areas of the body. Lay a hand gently over the heart, letting it be passive and receptive as if to acknowledge and cherish the heart's emotional vulnerability.

MELTING AND MERGING

While making love, there will be moments of blissful surrender to high orgasmic vibrations which move through your body like a current of electricity. Then there will be a time for tears, laughter, play and vulnerability as you relax and open yourselves to a whole range of human emotions. Periods of stillness and calm will take you into a deep and mysterious abyss as you dissolve into the sexual union. Lie together in silence so that your bodies fold into each other to have maximum skin contact. Again, move only enough to ensure the penis remains inside the vagina. Positions of melting and merging can include the man lying over the woman's back, or the woman, on top, yielding herself front-to-front to his body. In another position, the man can lie cupped behind his lover's body, placing his hand over her belly.

Breathe softly and in harmony, allowing yourselves to merge as one body and being. Let massage and making love lead you on a journey into the mysteries of sex.

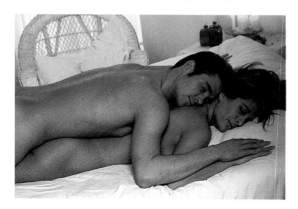

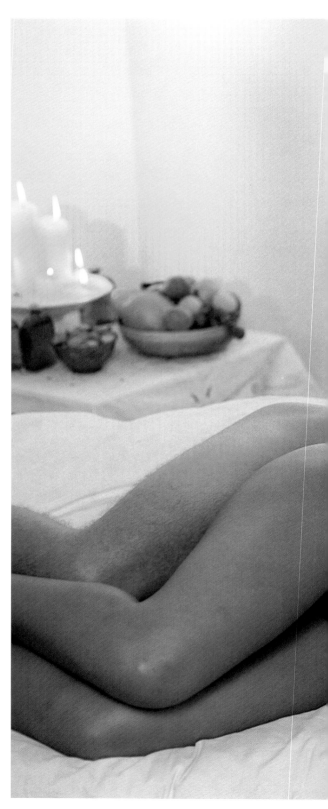

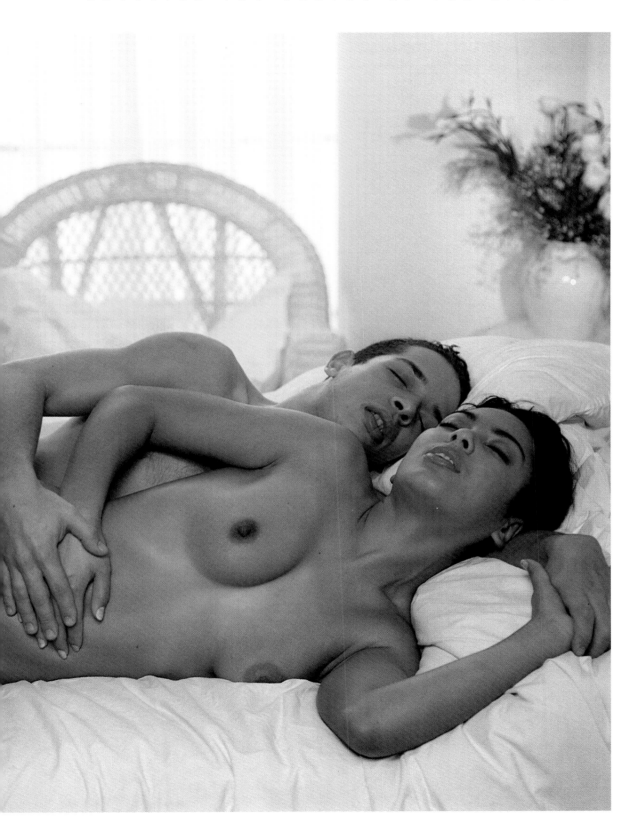

INDEX